ALL ABOUT NONPRESCRIPTION
DRUGS &
VITAMINS

SHEILA BUFF

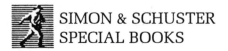

SIMON & SCHUSTER
SPECIAL BOOKS

IMPORTANT NOTICE

This book is intended only as a guide to nonprescription drugs used for medical self-treatment on the responsibility of the individual. It is not intended as a replacement for sound medical advice from a physician. This book does not contain every possible side effect, adverse or allergic reaction, or interaction with other drugs or substances. The final decision to self-treat a medical problem or to use a nonprescription drug rests with the individual in consultation with his or her physician. All recommendations herein are made without guarantees on the part of the author or the publisher. The author and the publisher disclaim all liability in connection with the use of this information.

The listing of selected brand names in this book is for ease of reference only. The inclusion of a brand name does not mean that the author or publisher has any particular knowledge that the brand listed has properties different from other brands of the same nonprescription drug. The inclusion of a brand name nonprescription drug should not be interpreted as an endorsement by the author or publisher. Similarly, that a brand name nonprescription drug is not included does not mean that the product is unsatisfactory or unacceptable. The author and the publisher disclaim all liability in connection with the use of this information.

Published by Simon & Schuster Special Books

Produced by Anthony Meisel Publishing Services
227 Park Avenue
Hoboken, NJ 07030

Printed in the United States of America

ISBN 0-671-79844-8

CONTENTS

INTRODUCTION

Life is full of aches and pains and minor ailments—colds, upset stomachs, head-aches, and the like. You can treat many of these problems easily and inexpensively by yourself using the convenient nonprescription medications readily available at drug stores. However, to use these products effectively and safely, you must understand what they are and how to take them—and when not to take them. In other words, you must be responsible for your self-medication.

Responsible self-medication is the informed and appropriate use of nonprescription medicines for the relief of symptoms, as well as the treatment, prevention and cure of certain conditions, on your own without the supervision of a health professional.

WHAT ARE NONPRESCRIPTION DRUGS?

Nonprescription drugs (also called over-the-counter drugs) are medicines available under law to the general public without a prescription. Federal law states that nonprescription drugs must be effective for their intended uses and must provide an appropriate margin of safety when used as directed. Label directions must be written in understandable language and must provide the information necessary for safe and effective use by the consumer. Nonprescription drugs cannot contain any drugs that are habit-forming or unsafe for use without a doctor's supervision.

Nonprescription medicines are widely recommended by doctors and dentists for self-treatment after they have diagnosed your problem. For example, once a doctor has diagnosed an ulcer, he or she may recommend nonprescription antacids instead of more expensive prescription medicines.

It is your responsibility as the consumer to read and understand nonprescription drug labels and to use these products properly. If you have any questions about any drug, ask your doctor, nurse, or pharmacist.

YOU AND YOUR PHARMACIST

Pharmacists (druggists) are licensed health-care professionals who dispense prescription and nonprescription medications in pharmacies (drug stores) and hospitals. Pharmacists are highly trained. They have college degrees in pharmacology and have passed rigorous certification examinations. They are very knowledgeable—often more knowledgeable than doctors—about the ingredients in *all* drugs. It is a pharmacist's job to provide information and counseling along with any medication, prescription or not. Never hesitate to ask for a pharmacist's help in selecting a nonprescription product or understanding how to use it.

To help you select the product that is most appropriate for you, a pharmacist will ask you questions about your general health as well as the specific problem. Be sure to mention any health problems or allergies you may have and any prescription or nonprescription products you use regularly. If you are or think might be pregnant, or if you are breast-feeding, be sure to tell the pharmacist. Sometimes a pharmacist may have to ask you somewhat intimate questions.

Answer honestly and try not to feel embarrassed; pharmacists follow the same confidentiality rules as doctors.

READING DRUG LABELS

The information you need to use a nonprescription drug properly and safely without professional supervision is on the label. In fact, the label of a nonprescription products contains much more information than the label of a prescription drug. By federal law, the label on each nonprescription medicine must include:

- The name and identity of the product.
- What the product will do.
- The net contents of the container.
- The active ingredients.
- The inactive ingredients.
- The name and location of the manufacturer, distributor, or packer.

The label must also include directions for using the product, including:

- The amount of each dose.
- How to take or apply the product.
- How often to take it.

The label must also include warnings about the product, including:

- The limits on use, if any.
- Side effects (drowsiness, for example), if any.
- Circumstances which may require a doctor's advice before taking the medicine (a preexisting health problem such as high blood pressure, for example).
- When to stop taking the medicine and see your doctor if the problem has not improved or has gotten worse.

Always check a nonprescription drug label for "flags." These are notices that inform you of a change in the product. For example, a flag might say "See side panel for new ingredients."

The label also includes an expiration number and a lot or batch code (sometimes this information is stamped on the crimp at the bottom of medicines in tubes). Never use a medicine that is past its expiration date—discard it safely instead. The lot or batch number helps the manufacturer trace the product if there is a problem with it.

AVOIDING DRUG INTERACTIONS

The label of any nonprescription drug includes detailed information about possible drug interactions. Some nonprescription products should not be used with certain prescription drugs (antacids should not be used with some prescription antibiotics, for example). If an unwanted interaction is possible between different medicines, the label will say so. If you regularly take any prescription or nonprescription drug, read this part of the label carefully. If you have any questions, ask your doctor or pharmacist.

Some nonprescription drugs also contain sodium. If the sodium content is higher than 5 mg per dose, the label says so. This is so that people who should restrict their intake of sodium can avoid or limit their use of the product.

In addition to the active ingredients, nonprescription drugs often contain inactive ingredients such as binders, fillers, and preservatives. Some nonprescription drugs also contain alcohol. All the inactive ingredients in a nonprescription product are listed on the label. This is so that people who may be allergic to an inactive ingredient or who should restrict their intake of alcohol or some other inactive ingredient can avoid or limit their use of the product.

PREGNANCY AND NURSING

Certain nonprescription drug labels must advise women who are pregnant or breast-feeding to seek the advice of a health professional before using the product. This is because some drugs may reach the fetus through the placenta or reach the baby through the mother's breast milk. If you are or think you may be pregnant, or if you are breast-feeding, read the label of any nonprescription product carefully before using it. If you have any questions at all about using the product, consult your doctor or pharmacist.

SEE YOUR DOCTOR

Nonprescription drugs are not always the answer to a health problem. The labels on most nonprescription drugs tell you when to see a doctor if your condition does not improve. In general, if your symptoms do not improve or get worse within a few days, see your doctor as soon as possible. A persistent problem can be a symptom of a more serious condition that needs medical attention. Be sure to tell your doctor about whatever nonprescription medications and other steps you have taken to self-treat the problem. Also be sure to tell your doctor about any other nonprescription and prescription drugs you take.

TAMPER-RESISTANT PACKAGING

The makers of nonprescription drugs seal their products in tamper-resistant packaging. This helps protect the consumer against possible criminal tampering. The type of tamper-resistant packaging used is always described on the label. Read the description carefully and check to make sure that the package has not been opened or damaged in any way. Don't purchase a package that looks as if it has been opened, damaged, or tampered with in any way. To help protect others, show damaged or suspicious packages to the pharmacist or store manager.

When you open the package, inspect the medicine itself. If it seems suspicious in any way, do not use the product. Look especially for capsules or tablets that are different in any way from the others in the package. Return suspicious products to the point of purchase as soon as possible.

If a product is packaged in a blister pack or other unit-dose package that cannot be reclosed, check every dose carefully before taking it.

KEEP OUT OF REACH OF CHILDREN

Young children can accidentally take nonprescription medicines—even those that taste bad to adults. Almost all nonprescription medicine labels have a warning that says: *"Keep this and all drugs out of the reach of children. In case of accidental overdose, seek professional assistance or contact your poison control center immediately."*

A list of poison control centers is found at the back of this book. If there is a poison control center near you, make a note of the phone number and keep it near the telephone along with other important emergency numbers.

Many nonprescription medicines are sold in containers with child safety closures. These caps are very effective, but they are no substitute for keeping the medicine out of the reach of children.

Household pets can accidentally ingest nonprescription medicines. A single acetaminophen tablet can kill a cat. Be sure to close all drug containers tightly. Find and discard any dropped tablets or capsules.

TAKING YOUR MEDICINE

The dosage for nonprescription medicines is listed on the label. Follow the directions. Do not take more of the medicine or take it more frequently unless your doctor specifically tells you otherwise.

Many liquid nonprescription medicines now come with "dose cups" to help you take the correct amount. Use the dose cup instead of ordinary spoons or cups from the kitchen. When taking other medications that require measuring, use standard measuring cups or spoons.

If you forget to take a dose on schedule, you can usually take it as soon as you remember. If you take a dose late, wait the recommended time between doses before taking the next. In general, do not double the next dose if you forget a dose completely.

Some nonprescription medicines will specifically state on the label that they should be taken with meals to lessen stomach irritation. Sometimes other specific information about taking the drug will be on the label. Read and follow these directions.

Many nonprescription drugs are in pill form as tablets or capsules. Some people have difficulty swallowing pills. If so, you can usually crush the tablet or open the capsule and sprinkle the powder on food or liquid. If a tablet or caplet is too large to swallow comfortably, try breaking it in half and taking each half separately. Do not, however, break up timed-release or long-lasting medications. Some medications are available in a variety of dose forms. Ask your pharmacist for help in selecting the product with the dose form you prefer.

SIDE EFFECTS

Some nonprescription medicines may have unwanted side effects. For example, aspirin can relieve headache pain but may cause nausea; antihistamines can relieve allergy sympotms but may cause drowsiness. Warnings about possible side effects are listed on the labels of nonprescription drugs. Your pharmacist or doctor can help you decide if the possible side effects outweigh the possible benefits of a nonprescription drug.

OVERDOSES AND ALLERGIC REACTIONS

Nonprescription drugs are generally safe to use without medical supervision in part because they do not contain large amounts of active ingredients. Even so, overdoses and allergic reactions may occur with these products.

Overdoses (accidental or otherwise) and severe allergic reactions are potentially dangerous or even life-threatening. Take immediate action:

• If the victim is unconscious and not breathing, shout for help. Do not leave the victim. Begin mouth-to-mouth respiration at once. Begin cardiopulmonary resuscitation (CPR) if it is needed and if you know how. Do not try to make the victim vomit.

• If the victim is unconscious but breathing, call 911 or 0 for emergency medical help. Do not try to make the victim vomit.

• If the victim is drowsy or semiconscious, call 911 or 0 for emergency medical help or take the victim to a nearby emergency room. Do not try to make the victim vomit.

• If the victim is alert, call 911 or 0 for emergency medical help, take the victim to a nearby emergency room, or call your local poison control center for instructions. Do not try to make the victim vomit unless you are told to do so.

• If the victim has no symptoms but you think an overdose has occurred, call your doctor or local poison control center for instructions.

A list of poison control centers is found at the back of this book. If there is a poison control center near you, make a note of the phone number and keep it near the telephone along with other important emergency numbers.

In all overdose and allergic reaction cases, always save the medicine container and all its contents. This will help medical workers determine how much of what medication was taken. If the victim vomits, save the vomit for analysis.

If an allergic reaction to a nonprescription drug is minor (rash, hives, or the like), stop using the product and call your doctor for instructions.

SYRUP OF IPECAC

Syrup of ipecac is a drug that induces vomiting. In some cases of overdose or accidental poisoning, you may be instructed to make the victim vomit by giving syrup of ipecac. One-ounce bottles of syrup of ipecac are available without prescription at pharmacies. A bottle should be kept securely in every home, particularly those with children. Use syrup of ipecac to induce vomiting *only* on medical advice.

TAKING DRUGS SAFELY

Never take *any* medicine in the dark. Keep all medications in their original containers with the original labels. Always check the label before taking any drug to make sure you are taking the correct medication in the correct way. Wear your eyeglasses when reading the label!

If you know you are allergic to a particular drug, read the label carefully to make sure the drug is not contained in the product. The label will often have warnings about possible allergic reactions.

Never take a prescription drug that has been prescribed for someone else, even if that person's symptoms are similar to yours.

STORING DRUGS

The traditional place to store medicines is the medicine cabinet in the bathroom, but few places could be worse. The bathroom can get hot and humid. In addition, children can often easily gain access to the medicine cabinet, which could lead to an accidental overdose. Store medicines in a cool, dry place that can be securely closed and is away from direct light. Do not store medicine in the refrigerator unless the label specifically tells you to. Keep liquid medicines from freezing. Always check the label of a medicine for additional storage information.

Check the contents of your medicine storage area regularly. Safely discard any old prescription medications that are no longer needed. Safely discard any nonprescription medicines that have passed their expiration date.

BRAND NAMES AND GENERIC DRUGS

All drugs, both prescription and nonprescription, have nonproprietary or "generic" names. Manufacturers give their own proprietary or "brand" names to the particular product they make using that generic drug. For example, the drug known by the generic name acetaminophen is the active ingredient in the drug know by the brand name Tylenol.

Many well-known nonprescription brand-name products are also available as generic products (also called no-name products or "house" brands). In general, when the ingredients lists of these products are compared, the generic versions are identical to the brand-name products. The difference is often in the cost— generic products are usually less expensive because they are not heavily advertised. Ask your pharmacist for help when comparing generic and brand-name products.

NONPRESCRIPTION DRUGS AND THE FDA

The Food and Drug Administration (FDA) is the federal agency responsible for determining the safety and effectiveness of all drugs, including nonprescription products. In 1972, the FDA began reviewing and evaluating all the nonprescription drugs sold in the United States. The goal of the ongoing study is to ensure that modern standards of science are applied and to ensure that these medicines are safe, effective, and properly labeled for consumer use without medical supervision. In some cases, the FDA has raised serious safety concerns. The drug industry has responded by removing some products from the market or by reformulating them to be safer.

On the other hand, the FDA has found that some drugs that were previously available only by doctor's prescription are safe for nonprescription use. Some examples of products that have been "switched" to nonprescription use are loperamide for diarrhea, ibuprofen for pain relief, clotrimazole for fungal infections, and many others. In fact, more than 200 nonprescription drugs today use ingredients or dosages available only by prescription in 1976.

THE SAVINGS TO YOU

When a drug is switched to nonprescription status, consumers benefit greatly. Currently 6 out of 10 medicines purchased by consumers are nonprescription products, yet total spending for these medications takes only 2 cents out of every health-care dollar.

In general, nonprescription products cost less. In addition, because you do not need a prescription to obtain them, nonprescription products save you the time and expense of a visit to the doctor's office. And because many drug stores are open late or even all night, you can purchase nonprescription drugs conveniently when you need them.

Remember, you are in charge of your own health. When using nonprescription drugs for self-treatment, be informed and be responsible.

ACNE

When Do You Need an Acne Product?

Acne products are widely used to treat the pimples and skin eruptions of common acne (acne vulgaris). Acne is an almost universal condition for adolescents, but acne occurs in young adults and in older persons as well. Acne can also be caused by cosmetics, high humidity, sweating, skin irritation or friction, and sometimes as a side effect of some prescription drugs.

Common acne in young people is usually caused by the hormonal changes of puberty. The increased hormonal activity leads to increased production of sebum (oil) by the sebaceous glands of the face and sometimes back and shoulders. The opening of the gland (pore) becomes clogged with sebum. As more sebum is secreted, the gland becomes enlarged and a whitehead becomes visible. In some cases, the plug of sebum protrudes above the skin surface. Sometimes the tip of the plug darkens to form a blackhead.

If the acne is limited to whiteheads and blackheads, it is known as noninflammatory acne. If, however, the whiteheads and blackheads often become inflamed or filled with pus, the condition is known as inflammatory acne. Noninflammatory acne can usually be controlled with good hygiene and nonprescription acne products. Inflammatory acne and severe noninflammatory acne should be treated by a doctor.

USING ACNE PRODUCTS

Noninflammatory acne can benefit from nonprescription products designed to help cleanse the face of excess sebum and dry lesions. The first step in controlling acne is good hygiene to remove excess sebum. Wash your face with soap and warm water. Pat the skin dry with a towel. Scrubbing hard while washing or drying may actually make acne worse. Ordinary soap without moisturizers or fragrances is usually effective. Acne formulations in soap are relatively ineffective, since the soap and any medication it contains is rinsed off. Cleansing pads with an alcohol base are helpful when washing with soap and water is inconvenient. Abrasive soaps and sponges can be helpful in cases of noninflammatory acne, but should be avoided in inflammatory acne. Some abrasive cleansing formulations contain polyethylene granules. Be careful not to get these products in the eyes. If an abrasive cleanser does get in the eyes, rinse thoroughly with clean water.

After cleansing, the next step in acne control is treating individual lesions. Topically applied acne medications can be effective for keeping pores open and unclogging blocked pores. Apply the product by spreading a small amount of it over the affected area once or twice daily. Acne medications should not be used near the eyes, mouth, lips, or inside the nose. These medications are for external use only.

Cleansers for acne come in a variety of forms, including bars, lotions, liquids, pads, and creams. Topical acne formulations also come in a variety of forms, including lotions, creams, ointments, gels, and sticks. Your choice of acne product will depend on the active ingredients you prefer and the form that is most convenient for you. Your pharmacist can help you select the brand that is most appropriate for you.

TYPES OF ACNE PRODUCTS

Benzoyl Peroxide

Benzoyl peroxide is a very effective nonprescription treatment for common acne. It helps keep pores open, helps open clogged pores, and helps dry lesions. It may also help kill bacteria that can lead to infection.

Benzoyl peroxide products are usually available in 2.5 percent, 5 percent, and 10 percent concentrations. The numbers 5 and 10 often appear in the brand names of products that contain benzoyl peroxide in those concentrations. If a higher concentration product dries the skin too much, try a lower concentration.

Benzoyl peroxide occasionally stings or burns slightly on application. The sensation usually passes quickly. However, some people are sensitive to benzoyl peroxide. Symptoms of sensitivity include itching, burning, redness, and swelling around the affected area. If sensitivity develops, stop using the product.

Sulfur

Sulfur is an effective nonprescription treatment for common acne, particularly for helping blemishes to clear. Sulfur acne products usually contain sulfur, zinc sulfide, or sodium thiosulfate. A major drawback to sulfur products is their distinct color and odor.

Salicylic Acid

Salicylic acid is an acceptable nonprescription treatment for acne, although it is not as effective as benzoyl peroxide or sulfur. Salicylic acid is found in many acne products that also contain alcohol. The alcohol probably does more to help the acne. Salicylic acid may be harmful if it is extensively used for a long time.

Resorcinol

Some nonprescription acne products contain resorcinol. By itself resorcinol is not effective for treating acne. In combination with other acne medications, it does no harm.

Combination Products

Some acne formulations combine ingredients such as salicylic acid and sulfur. These formulations may be slightly more effective than the individual ingredients alone.

Other Ingredients

Many liquid acne medications and cleansing formulations contain alcohol. Because alcohol has a drying effect on the skin, it is often helpful. When the active ingredients in the product are salicylic acid or resorcinol, the alcohol is often the most beneficial ingredient in the formulation.

Acne formulations can contain a variety of preservatives, coloring agents, fragrances, and other ingredients. Generally these ingredients are harmless, but some people may be sensitive to some of them. If you are not sensitive to benzoyl peroxide, and if an acne product burns, itches, makes your skin red, or makes your blemishes worse, stop using it. Try a different brand instead.

SPECIAL CONSIDERATIONS

Children: Do not use an acne product for skin blemishes on children.

Acne Product Cautions

Possible side effects: Some people are sensitive to benzoyl peroxide. If a reaction develops, stop using the product.

Call Your Doctor:

• If you have severe noninflammatory acne.

• If you have inflammatory acne.

• If a blemish becomes infected or develops an abscess.

• If you think your acne is a result of a prescription drug.

ACNE PRODUCTS AND COMMON BRANDS

BENZOYL PEROXIDE PRODUCT	
Brand Name	*Application Form*
Acne-Aid	cream
Ben-Aqua 5	lotion
Ben-Aqua 10	lotion
Benoxyl 5	lotion
Benoxyl 10	lotion
Clear By Design	gel
Clearasil Benzoyl Peroxide	cream, lotion
Cuticura Acne Cream	cream
Del Aqua-5	gel
Del Aqua-10	gel
Dry and Clear	cream, lotion
Fostex 5% BPO	gel
Fostex 10% BPO	bar, cream, gel, cleanser
Fostril	lotion
Loroxide	lotion
Neutrogena Acne Mask	clay mask
Noxzema Clear-Ups	lotion
Noxzema On-the-Spot Treatment	lotion
Oxy-5	lotion
Oxy-10	lotion
PanOxyl Bar 5	cleanser
PanOxyl Bar 10	cleanser
pHisoAc BP	cream
Propa P.H. Liquid Acne Soap	liquid
Stri-Dex Maximum Strength	cream
Vanoxide	lotion
Xerac BP 10	gel
Xerac BP 10	gel

SULFUR PRODUCTS

Brand Name	Application Form
Acnederm	lotion
Acno Lotion	lotion
Acnophill	ointment
Buf-Bar	bar
Cuticura	ointment
Finac Lotion	lotion
Fostex Medicated Cover-Up	cream
Liquimat	lotion
Lotio Alsulfa	lotion
Seale's Lotion Modified	lotion
Sulfur Soap	cleanser
Sulpho-Lac	cleanser
Sulray	bar, cream
Xerac Alcohol Gel	gel
Zinc Sulfide Compound Lotion, Improved	lotion

SALICYLIC ACID PRODUCTS

Brand Name	Application Form
Aveeno Cleansing Bar	bar
Clear By Design	pads
Clearasil Double Clear Pads	pads
Clearasil Medicated Astringent	liquid
Drytex Lotion	lotion
Ionax Astringent Skin Cleanser	liquid
Komed	lotion
Listerex Golden Lotion	abrasive cleanser
Listerex Herbal Lotion	abrasive cleanser
Medicated Face Conditioner	liquid
Noxzema Clear-Ups Anti-Acne Gel	gel
Noxzema Clear-Ups Medicated Skin Cleansing Pads	pads
Oxy Clean Maximum Strength Cleanser	cleanser
Oxy Clean Maximum Strength Pads	pads
Oxy Clean Medicated Cleanser	cleanser
Oxy Clean Medicated Pads	pads
Oxy Clean Medicated Soap	soap
Propa P.H. Medicated with Aloe	pads, cream, stick
SalAc Cleanser	liquid
Salicylic Acid Soap	bar
Saligel Acne Gel	gel
Stri-Dex Lotion	lotion
Stri-Dex Maximum Strength Medicated	pads
Stri-Dex Medicated	pads

SULFUR WITH SALICYLIC ACID/RESORCINOL

Brand Name	Application Form
Acnomel	cream
Acnotex	lotion
Bensulfoid	cream
Clearasil Adult Care	cream, stick
Fostex Medicated Cleansing Bar	bar
Pernox Lotion	lotion
Pernox Regular	abrasive cleanser
Pernox Lemon	abrasive cleanser
pHisoAc	cream
Rezamid	lotion
Salicylic Acid and Sulfur Soap	bar
Sastid Plain Therapeutic Wash	cleanser
Sastid Soap	cleanser
Sebasorb	liquid
Therac	lotion

CLEANSING PRODUCTS

Brand Name	Application Form
Acne-Aid Cleansing Bar	bar
Acno Cleanser	liquid
Betadine Skin Cleanser	cleanser
Brasivol	abrasive cleanser
Brasivol Base	liquid
Clearasil Antibacterial Bar	soap
Ionax Foam	foam
Ionax Scrub	abrasive cleanser
Komex	abrasive cleanser
Noxzema Antiseptic Skin Cleanser Regular Strength	cleanser
Noxzema Antiseptic Skin Cleanser Extra Strength	cleanser
Noxzema Antiseptic Skin Cleanser Sensitive Skin	cleanser
Oxy Wash	cleanser
Seba-Nil	solution
Seba-Nil Cleansing Mask	abrasive cleanser
Tyrosum Packets	cleanser

ANTACIDS

When Do You Need an Antacid?

Antacids are widely used to relieve the occasional symptoms of heartburn, indigestion, "sour stomach," gastritis, and discomfort from overindulgence in food or drink. Under medical supervision, antacids are also used to control the long-term symptoms of peptic ulcer and reflux esophagitis.

USING ANTACIDS

The active ingredients in antacids neutralize gastric acid. Some antacids also contain ingredients that relieve gas symptoms.

Many antacids are high in sodium (often in the form of sodium bicarbonate), even though many brands have been reformulated in recent years to reduce their sodium content. If an antacid contains more than 5 mg of sodium per dosage unit, the label of the container will indicate this. If you should restrict your intake of sodium, read the container label carefully and consult your pharmacist about which product is best for you.

Some antacids contain aspirin or bismuth, which is a salicylate related to aspirin. If you are hypersensitive to aspirin, do not use an antacid containing aspirin or bismuth. (For more information about aspirin hypersensitivity, see the section on pain relievers.)

In addition to the active ingredients and the ingredients mentioned above, some antacids also contain acetaminophen, citric acid, glycine, mint flavoring, saccharin, sorbitol, or sugar. If you should restrict your intake of any of these ingredients, consult your pharmacist about which product is best for you.

Antacids come as liquids, suspensions, gels, chewable tablets, effervescent tablets, tablets, capsules, granules, powders, and even chewing gum. Your choice of antacid will depend on the active ingredients you prefer, the flavoring you prefer, and the form you prefer to take them in. Liquids and suspensions are by far the most effective way to take antacids because the particles of active ingredient are already very fine. The finer the particles, the more excess stomach acid they can absorb. By contrast, the particles in tablets and chewable tablets are much bigger and absorb less acid. On a comparative basis, then, it takea many more chewable tablets to equal the same effect as one dose of liquid antacid. When using effervescent antacid tablets, dissolve the tablets in water and wait until most of the bubbles are gone before drinking.

Not all antacids are equally potent at the same dosage level. The neutralizing capacity of different antacids depends on their formulation. The 5 most effective liquid antacids, in descending order, are Maalox TC, Mylanta II, Delcid, Titralac, and Camalox. The 5 most effective tablet antacids, in descending order, are Camalox, Basaljel, Mylanta II, Tums, and Alka II.

The neutralizing effects of antacids generally last about 30 minutes when taken on an empty stomach. When taken 1 hour after a meal, the neutralizing effect of antacids generally last about 3 hours.

Unless your doctor recommends antacids on an ongoing basis, stop taking antacids when your symptoms subside. Do not take antacids for the relief of indigestion for longer than 2 weeks.

TYPES OF ANTACIDS

Sodium Bicarbonate

Sodium bicarbonate (also called baking soda or bicarb) is a well-known and very effective home remedy for the occasional relief of mild indigestion and the symptoms of eating or drinking too much. It is easily prepared at home by dissolving 1/2 teaspoon sodium bicarbonate in 4 fluid ounces of water. Sodium bicarbonate is high in sodium and should be avoided by people who should restrict their sodium intake. Sodium bicarbonate can react with milk or calcium in the diet to cause milk-alkali syndrome. Do not take sodium bicarbonate on a regular basis.

Calcium Carbonate

Antacids containing calcium have the greatest effect. Calcium carbonate is the active ingredient in most calcium-containing antacids.

Magnesium

Antacids containing magnesium salts generally use magnesium hydroxide, magnesium carbonate, or magnesium oxide. Magnesium has less neutralizing ability than sodium bicarbonate or calcium carbonate, but more than aluminum. Antacids containing magnesium should not be used by people with kidney problems.

Aluminum

Antacids containing aluminum generally use aluminum hydroxide, although aluminum phosphate or aluminum carbonate are sometimes used. Of the forms of aluminum used, aluminum hydroxide is the most effective for neutralizing stomach acid. Aluminum has less neutralizing ability than sodium bicarbonate, calcium carbonate, or magnesium. Antacids containing aluminum alone can cause constipation.

Magnesium-Aluminum Combinations

Antacids containing magnesium and aluminum in combination are about as effective as either ingredient alone.

Simethicone

Simethicone is an inert substance that has a defoaming effect—that is, it breaks up gas bubbles in the stomach. This helps relieve symptoms and allows the gas to be passed more easily. Simethicone is found in many antacid formulations. Although simethicone does not work well in the presence of aluminum, some antacid formulations contain both ingredients. If gas is the primary symptom, select an antacid that contains simethicone but not aluminum. Your pharmacist can help you select the brand that is best for you.

Bismuth

Bismuth is an effective liquid antacid. However, bismuth contains salicylate and can cause dangerous allergic reactions in people who are hypersensitive to aspirin. A harmless side effect of bismuth is temporary blackening of the stool and occasionally of the tongue.

Alginic Acid

Alginic acid is used to help prevent the uncomfortable symptoms caused by esophagal reflux and hiatus hernia. It is not an antacid. Use alginic acid only on the recommendation of your physician. When a tablet containing alginic acid and sodium bicarbonate is chewed, swallowed, and followed by a large glass of water, a harmless foam is formed in the stomach. The foam floats on top of the gastric contents. If a reflux occurs, the foam, not the stomach acids, comes in contact with the esophagus. In mild to moderate cases, this helps prevent discomfort, pain, and heartburn.

SPECIAL CONSIDERATIONS

Children: Because of the risk of Reye's syndrome, do not give children an antacid containing bismuth.

Pregnant and nursing women: Avoid antacids, particularly those containing sodium.

Elderly persons: Antacids that can cause constipation or diarrhea are more likely to have these effects on elderly people.

Antacid Overdose

An overdose of an antacid is unlikely to be life-threatening. Get medical advice if a overdose occurs. An overdose of simethicone is unlikely to cause problems.

Cautions for Antacids

Possible side effects: In general antacids have side effects only if taken in large quantities for a long time. Side effects of antacids can include constipation, diarrhea, headache, and distended stomach. Simethicone is unlikely to have side effects.

Possible drug interactions: Do not take antacids if you take a medication containing chlorpromazine. Antacids will decrease the effectiveness of tetracycline, penicillin, some other antibiotics, and indomethican. Wait at least 3 hours after taking the drug to take an antacid. Discuss dosing intervals with your pharmacist if you take any prescription drug. Avoid antacids if you take medication containing digitalis or medication for a heart rhythm disorder. Antacids strongly increase the effectiveness of levodopa. Take antacids with this drug only with the advice of your physician.

Other medical problems: Avoid antacids containing sodium or magnesium if you have kidney disease. Avoid antacids containing sodium if you have high blood pressure, congestive heart failure, edema, or are pregnant.

Call Your Doctor:

- If your symptoms do not get better after taking antacids for 2 weeks.
- If you vomit blood or black material that resembles coffee grounds.
- If you have severe abdominal pain.
- If you have a burning or gnawing pain in the abdomen or chest.
- If your stool contains blood or is black or tarry.

ANTACIDS AND COMMON BRANDS

CALCIUM CARBONATE	
Brand Name	*Dose Form*
Algenic Alka	liquid
Alka-Mints	chewable tablet
Amitone	tablet
Calcilac	tablet
Calcium Carbonate	tablet, suspension
Calglycine	chewable tablet

Chooz	chewing gum*
Diatrol	tablet
Dicarbosil	tablet
Dimacid	chewable tablet
Equilet	chewable tablet
Genalac	chewable tablet
Glycate	tablet
Mallamint	chewable tablet
Marblen	tablet, suspension
Noralac	chewable tablet
Rolaids Calcium Rich	chewable tablet
Spastosed	tablet
Titracid	chewable tablet
Titralac	chewable tablet
Titralac Plus	liquid**
Tums	chewable tablet
Tums Extra Strength	liquid
Tums E-X Extra Strength	chewable tablet
	* sodium free
	** contains simethicone

ALUMINUM HYDROXIDE

Brand Name	*Dose Form*
Algicon	chewable tablet
ALternaGel	suspension**
Alu-Cap	capsule
Aluminum Hydroxide (generic)	tablet, suspension, gel
Alu-Tab	tablet
Amphojel	tablet, suspension
Dialume	tablet
Duracid	chewable tablet
Gaviscon ESRF	suspension
Nephrox	suspension
Phosphaljel	suspension
	** contains simethicone

MAGNESIUM OXIDE OR HYDROXIDE

Brand Name	*Dose Form*
Mag-Ox 400	tablet*
Maox	tablet
Milk of Magnesia (generic)	tablet, suspension
Phillips' Milk of Magnesia	tablet, suspension
Rolaids Sodium Free	chewable tablet
Uro-Mag	capsule*
	* sodium free

ALUMINUM/MAGNESIUM COMBINATION

Brand Name	Dose Form
Algenic Alka Improved	chewable tablet
Almacone	chewable tablet, suspension**
Almacone II	suspension**
Alma-Mag Improved	liquid**
Alma-Mag #4 Improved	chewable tablet**
Aludrox	suspension**
Anta Gel	liquid**
Anta Gel II	liquid**
Banacid	chewable tablet
Creamalin	tablet
Di-Gel	liquid*,**
Gelusil	chewable tablet, liquid*,**
Gelusil II	chewable tablet, liquid*,**
Kessadrox	suspension
Kolantyl	gel
Kudrox Double Strength	liquid
Liquid Antacid	liquid
Maalox	tablet, suspension
Maalox Extra Strength	tablet
Maalox Plus	tablet**
Maalox Plus Extra Strength	liquid, suspension**
Maalox TC	tablet, suspension
Magnagel	tablet
Magna Gel	suspension
Magnesia and Alumina Oral Suspension	suspension
Mi-Acid	liquid**
Mintox	suspension**
Mintox Plus	liquid**
Mygel	suspension**
Mylanta	tablet, suspension**
Mylanta II	tablet, suspension**
Rulox	suspension**
Rulox #1	chewable tablet
Rulox #2	chewable tablet
Simaal Gel	liquid**
Simaal 2 Gel	liquid**
Triconsil	chewable tablet
Trimagel	tablet
WinGel	tablet, suspension
	* sodium free
	** contains simethicone

CALCIUM WITH ALUMINUM AND/OR MAGNESIUM

Brand Name	Dose Form
Alamag	suspension
Alkets	tablet
Bicalma	chewable tablet
Camalox	tablet, suspension
Di-Gel Advanced Formula	chewable tablet**
Magnatril	chewable tablet, suspension
Tempo Drops	chewable tablet*,**
	* sodium free
	** contains simethicone

SIMETHICONE

Brand Name	Dose Form
Gas-X	chewable tablet*
Gas-X Extra Strength	chewable tablet*
Lowsium	chewable tablet, suspension
Lowsium Plus	tablet, suspension
Mylicon	chewable tablet
Mylicon Drops	drops
Mylicon-80	chewable tablet
Mylicon-125	chewable tablet
Riopan Plus	chewable tablet, suspension
Riopan Plus Extra Strength	chewable tablet, suspension
	* sodium free

SODIUM BICARBONATE

Brand Name	Dose Form
Alka-Seltzer Effervescent	effervescent tablet
Alka-Seltzer Extra Strength	effervescent tablet
Alka-Seltzer Flavored	effervescent tablet
Alka-Seltzer with Aspirin	effervescent tablet
Bell/ans	tablet
BiSoDol	tablet, powder
Bromo-Seltzer	granules
Citrocarbonate	granules

ALGINIC ACID

Brand Name	Dose Form
Gaviscon	chewable tablet, suspension
Gaviscon ESR	tablet
Gaviscon-2	chewable tablet

ASTHMA

When Do You Need an Asthma Medication?
Asthma medications help relieve the wheeziness, shortness of breath, and tightness in the chest of a mild asthma attack. The most common cause of asthma attacks is allergies, including seasonal allergies (pollen, for example), perennial allergies (house dust, for example), allergies to other substances (flour or industrial dust, for example), food allergies (shellfish or chocolate, for example), and sometimes drug allergies (aspirin, for example). Stress, air pollutants, respiratory tract infections, and exercise may also trigger asthma attacks. Nonprescription asthma medications contain bronchodilators, which help relax the bronchial passages of the lungs and relieve the symptoms of asthma.

USING ASTHMA MEDICATIONS

If you think you may have asthma, it is very important that you see your doctor before taking any nonprescription drugs to relieve the symptoms. In many cases asthma attacks are occasional and mild and respond well to nonprescription medications. However, asthma can be a serious condition, especially if you don't realize that you are having a severe attack or if you also have heart disease or high blood pressure. The symptoms of chronic bronchitis and emphysema are similar to those of asthma. Once your doctor diagnoses asthma, he or she may recommend a prescription drug or suggest a nonprescription medication. Nonprescription asthma medications contain bronchodilators, which help relieve the symptoms of mild asthma attacks. They do not treat the underlying cause of asthma attacks and do not keep the attacks from happening. Never exceed the recommended dose.

In addition to the active ingredients, a few aerosol asthma medications contain alcohol. If you are concerned about this, consult your pharmacist about which product is best for you.

USING INHALERS

Although some asthma medications come in tablet form and are swallowed, most nonprescription asthma medications are taken by breathing them into the lungs using an aerosol inhaler. The inhaler delivers a metered dose (usually 10, 15, or 20 ml) of the medication. One inhaler usually contains hundreds of doses. Your pharmacist can help you select the brand that is best for you.

For the maximum benefit, it is important to use the inhaler properly. Follow these simple steps: Shake the inhaler well. Place the mouthpiece between the lips and close your mouth around it, making sure to move your teeth and tongue out of the way. (An alternative but less effective method is to hold the inhaler about 1 inch in front of your open mouth.) Breathe out (exhale) slowly. Next, activate the inhaler while breathing in (inhaling) slowly and deeply. Hold your breath for at least 10 seconds, then exhale. If you need a second dose, wait at least 1 minute. Never exceed the recommended dose. If your symptoms are not relieved within 5 to 10 minutes, get medical help immediately.

Asthma sufferers sometimes think that an aerosol asthma medication isn't helping when in fact they are using it improperly. Your pharmacist can show you the correct method for using inhalers and answer your questions about them.

Some nonprescription asthma medications are meant to be used with a nebulizer, a hand-held device that uses a rubber bulb to spray the medication into the lungs. Your doctor or pharmacist can show you the correct way to make use of a nebulizer.

TYPES OF ASTHMA MEDICATIONS

Epinephrine

Epinephrine is the active ingredient in aerosol asthma medications. This drug is a bronchodilator that helps relieve wheezing, shortness of breath, and tightness in the chest. Epinephrine usually works within 5 to 10 minutes. Never exceed the recommended dosage.

Theophylline/Ephedrine Combination

On its own, theophylline is an effective bronchodilator that a doctor must pre-scribe for you. Ephedrine is also a bronchodilator but it is relatively ineffective. These drugs are often combined in tablet form. They are not as effective or fast-acting as epinephrine medications and should be used only for very mild asthma attacks. Because they are not inhaled, theophylline/ephedrine combination drugs take about 1 hour to reach their peak effect; relief lasts about 5 hours. Never exceed the recommended dosage.

Many theophylline/ephedrine combination drugs also contain phenobarbital. The sale of nonprescription drugs containing phenobarbital is restricted in many states; in addition, the value of phenobarbital has not been shown. Asthma medications containing phenobarbital are not discussed in this book, but your pharmacist can answer your questions about them.

Some theophylline/ephedrine combination drugs also contain guaifenesin (an expectorant). However, the value of guaifenesin has not been shown. Asthma medications containing guaifenesin are not discussed in this book, but your pharmacist can answer your questions about them.

SPECIAL CONSIDERATIONS

Children: Do not give asthma medications to children under the age of 4 except under the advice and supervision of a physician. Never exceed the recommended dose.

Pregnant and nursing women: Avoid asthma medications if you are pregnant. Asthma medications pass into milk. Avoid them if you are nursing or stop nurs-ing until you stop taking the medication. Never exceed the recommended dose.

Elderly persons: Asthma medications may lead to high blood pressure, heart-rhythm problems and angina. The stimulant effect may be felt more. Never exceed the recommended dose.

Asthma Medication Abuse

Asthma medications containing phenobarbital can be abused and may be habit-forming.

Asthma Medication Overdose

Symptoms of asthma medication overdose include rapid and irregular pulse, anxiety, muscle cramps, and chest pain. Get medical help immediately.

Cautions for Asthma Medications

Overuse: Many asthma sufferers overuse nonprescription medications. Overuse of epinephrine medications may cause rapid heartbeat and nervousness. Overuse of theophylline/ephedrine combinations may cause nervousness, insomnia, and nausea.

Possible side effects: Side effects of epinephrine and ephedrine include insomnia, nervousness, rapid heartbeat, difficulty in urination, muscle tremors, and nausea. If you use asthma medications only occasionally, these side effects will probably be minor. If you use asthma medications frequently, discuss the side effects with your doctor.

Possible drug interactions: Do not take asthma medications if you also take antidepressants, high blood pressure medications, MAO inhibitors, or drugs containing ergot. Do not take nonprescription asthma medications in addition to prescription asthma medications.

Other medical problems: Do not take asthma medications if you have high blood pressure, chronic pulmonary disease, heart disease, diabetes, thyroid disease, seizure disorder, or difficulty in urination due to an enlarged prostate gland.

Call Your Doctor:

• If you do not get prompt relief from inhaler treatment.
• If your symptoms become worse or more frequent.

ASTHMA MEDICATIONS AND COMMON BRANDS

EPINEPHRINE

Active Ingredient: Epinephrine

Brand Name	Dose Form
Adrenalin Chloride	nebulizer solution
AsthmaHaler	inhaler
AsthmaNefrin	nebulizer solution
Breatheasy	inhaler
Bronitin Mist	inhaler
Bronkaid Mist	inhaler
Bronkaid Mist Suspension	inhaler
Dey-Dose Epinephrine	nebulizer solution
Epinephrine (generic)	inhaler
Medihaler-Epi	inhaler
microNEFRIN	nebulizer solution
Primatene Mist Solution	inhaler
Primatene Mist Suspension	inhaler
S-2 Inhalant Solution	nebulizer solution
Vaponefrin	nebulizer solution

COMBINATION MEDICATIONS
Active Ingredients: Theophylline and Ephedrine

Brand Name	*Dose Form*
Amesec	capsule
Primatene	tablet
Primatene M	tablet
Primatene NS	tablet

ATHLETE'S FOOT AND OTHER FUNGAL INFECTIONS

When Do You Need an Antifungal Product?

Antifungal products help relieve and often cure the itching, redness, scaling, burning, blistering, and oozing of athlete's foot (tinea pedis). Antifungal products also help relieve and often cure the scaly, reddish, ring-shaped patches of ringworm (tinea corporis) and the itchy red lesions of "jock itch" (tinea cruris).

Fungal infections are very common. They thrive on those parts of the human body that are warm and moist, especially the feet and groin. Anyone of any age can get a fungal infection.

Athlete's foot is a fungal infection not at all confined to athletes. Although you are more likely to get athlete's foot if you regularly participate in sports that make your feet get sweaty inside closed shoes, you may also get athlete's foot simply because you wear leather shoes, synthetic socks, or nylon pantyhose. In general, athlete's foot can take one of three forms. The most common type of athlete's foot is a fungal infection usually found on the webbing between the fourth and fifth (little) toes. Symptoms include mild to severe itching, burning, scaling and sometimes cracking of the skin, and weeping or oozing. The symptoms sometimes spread to the sole or arch of the foot. Symptoms of the second type of athlete's foot are widespread dry scaling on the sides of the feet and the lower heel. The primary symptom of the third type of athlete's foot is small blisters between the toes; the blisters may spread to the bottom of the foot. The blisters rupture, leaving ragged, sore areas. The third type is more likely to occur in warm, humid weather.

The best treatment for athlete's foot is prevention. Good hygiene and keeping the feet dry are the most important preventive measures. Wash the feet daily with soap and water. Dry them thoroughly with a clean towel, being sure to dry between the toes. Let your feet air for 5 to 10 minutes before putting on socks, stockings or shoes. Some people find that a light dusting of talcum powder or cornstarch on the feet helps absorb moisture. If you feet sweat heavily, disposable, absorbent insoles placed in your shoes may help. Materials that do not breathe (nylon and other synthetic materials, for example) trap moisture on the feet, creating a breeding ground for fungus. Whenever possible, wear absorbent socks made of natural fiber and lightweight shoes that freely encourage air circulation.

Change shoes frequently so that moisture doesn't build up in them.

Athlete's foot is most common among men aged 14 and up. It is less common in women, but as more women become athletically active, the incidence is rising. Athlete's foot is not often seen in children. If a child develops symptoms similar to athlete's foot, a doctor should be consulted. If you have diabetes or circulatory problems, see your doctor if you develop the symptoms of athlete's foot.

Ringworm, despite its name, is a fungal infection. The primary symptoms of ringworm are scaly, reddish, itchy, ring-shaped patches with raised borders; in later stages, the patches may become inflamed and produce a red-hot burning sensation. The patches are generally about 1 inch across and may be found almost anywhere on the body. If ringworm develops on the scalp, patches of temporary baldness may occur.

Ringworm is most common in children, who may get it from other children or from household pets. Ringworm is contagious. A child with ringworm should stay home from school until the infection is over. If the ringworm is on the scalp, discard any combs, brushes, hats, and the like that the child may have used. Consult a doctor about treating ringworm in children; consult a doctor if an adult develops ringworm on the scalp or other hairy parts of the body.

"Jock itch" is caused by fungal infections, not by jock straps. However, any article of clothing that traps moisture or causes chafing in the delicate groin area may trigger the development of jock itch. Wet swimsuits and athletic wear made from spandex, lycra, nylon and other nonbreathing fabrics can be breeding grounds for the fungus that causes jock itch. The primary symptoms of jock itch are red, raised, itchy lesions on the inner upper thigh and the groin area. The lesions sometimes spread to the buttocks.

As with athlete's foot, good hygiene and keeping the area dry are the best preventive measures. Some people find that a light dusting of talcum powder or cornstarch on the groin helps absorb moisture. Wash athletic wear often and store it in an airy place—not a dark gym locker or bag.

USING ANTIFUNGALS

Nonprescription antifungal products contain ingredients that relieve the symptoms of athlete's foot, ringworm, and jock itch and also kill the fungi that cause the symptoms. A number of safe and effective ingredients are available.

Antifungals are usually found as creams, solutions, and powders. Solutions are available as aerosol and pump sprays. Powders are available in shaker containers and as aerosol and pump sprays. Creams should be applied as a thin layer directly over the affected area. Solutions are generally dabbed or sprayed onto the affected area, while powders are shaken or sprayed on.

In general, athlete's foot takes about 4 weeks to improve markedly or disappear altogether. Jock itch and ringworm usually take about 2 weeks to improve.

Your choice of antifungal will depend on the active ingredients you prefer and the application form that is most convenient for you. Your pharmacist can help you select the brand that is most appropriate for you.

TYPES OF ANTIFUNGALS

Clotrimazole

Clotrimazole is a very effective antifungal that has only recently become available on a nonprescription basis. It is effective for all types of athlete's foot, ringworm, and jock itch.

Miconazole Nitrate

Miconazole nitrate is an effective antifungal, particularly for jock itch and athlete's foot. Burning and irritation are occasional side effects.

Tolnaftate

Tolnaftate is an effective antifungal that is particularly helpful for the dry, scaling type of athlete's foot. Products containing tolnaftate usually sting slightly on application. It should be applied sparingly twice a day.

Undecylenic Acid/Zinc Undecylenate

Undecylenic acid, often combined with zinc undecylenate, is an effective treatment for athlete's foot, particularly the dry, scaling type.

Aluminum Acetate/Aluminum Chloride

Aluminum acetate solution (Burow's solution) and aluminum chloride solution do not cure athlete's foot. They are useful, however, for treating the wet, soggy tissue of severe athlete's foot, because they have an astringent effect that helps dry the affected area. Aluminum chloride may kill bacteria and help prevent secondary infection. For best results, soak the whole foot in the solution for 20 minutes 3 times daily.

Aluminum acetate and aluminum chloride are poisonous if swallowed. Keep these products away from children.

For more information about these products, see the section on poison ivy and poison oak.

Salicylic Acid

Some antifungal products contain salicylic acid as the primary ingredient. Salicylic acid is not considered safe and effective for treating athlete's foot and other fungal infections.

SPECIAL CONSIDERATIONS

Children: Consult your doctor about treating ringworm, athlete's foot, and other fungal infections.

Antifungal Cautions

Possible side effects: Miconazole nitrate may cause burning and itching. Tolnaftate usually stings slightly on application.

Other medical problems: Do not use nonprescription antifungals if you have diabetes, circulatory problems, or another infection.

Call Your Doctor:

• If you have diabetes and develop symptoms of athlete's foot.

• If you have circulatory problems in your legs and develop symptoms of athlete's foot.

• If a child has ringworm or athlete's foot.

• If an adult has ringworm on the scalp or other hairy parts of the body.

- If your athlete's foot symptoms include white, soggy tissue, oozing, very severe itching, or foot odor.
- If you have a fungal infection of the fingernails or toenails.
- If your athlete's foot does not improve or gets worse after 4 weeks of treatment.
- If your ringworm or jock itch does not improve or gets worse after 2 weeks.

ANTIFUNGAL MEDICATIONS AND COMMON BRANDS

CLOTRIMAZOLE PRODUCTS

Brand Name	Application Form
Lotrimin AF	cream, solution
Mycelex OTC	cream, solution

TOLNAFTATE PRODUCTS

Brand Name	Application Form
Aftate	powder, gel, spray liquid, spray powder
Dr. Scholl's Athlete's Foot	cream, powder, spray liquid, spray powder
Genaspor	cream
NP-27	cream, powder, solution, spray powder
Odor-Eaters	cream
Tinactin	cream, powder, solution, spray powder, spray liquid
Ting	cream, powder, spray powder, spray liquid
Tritin	powder
Zeasorb-AF	powder

MICONAZOLE NITRATE

Brand Name	Application Form
Micatin	cream, powder, spray powder, spray liquid

UNDECYLENIC ACID/ZINC UNDECYLENATE PRODUCTS

Brand Name	Application Form
Cruex	powder
Decylenes	ointment
Dermasept Antifungal	liquid
Desenex	cream, powder, ointment, soap, spray powder
Desenex Antifungal	foam
Desenex Liquid	solution
Deso-Creme	cream
Merlenate	ointment
Quinsana Plus Medicated	powder
Undoguent	ointment
Undecylenic Acid Compound (generic)	ointment

BURNS AND SUNBURN

When Do You Need a Burn or Sunburn Product?

Burn products help relieve the pain of first-degree burns and minor second-degree burns. Sunburn products help relieve the pain of minor to moderate sunburn.

Burns are one of the most common minor injuries. Most burn injuries occur in the home; many are related to cooking. Many minor burns in the household could be prevented by common sense and simple safety precautions: using potholders, keeping matches and lighters away from children, not smoking in bed (preferably not smoking at all), not leaving hot irons unattended, and so on. Many serious burn injuries and fire-related deaths could be prevented by having functioning smoke detectors in homes, schools, work places, and elsewhere. Smoke detectors are inexpensive and easy to install and maintain—and they can save your life.

Burns are classified by degree of severity. First-degree burns are minor burns affecting just the surface of the skin. These burns are red and painful, but the skin is not blistered. First-degree burns generally heal in 3 to 4 days and leave no scar. Second-degree burns are more serious because they affect the skin surface and the tissue just below it. Second-degree burns are characterized by redness, blisters, oozing, and more severe pain. Minor second-degree burns generally heal in about 3 weeks and leave no scar. Severe second-degree burns can take a month or more to heal and can leave thick scars. Third- and fourth-degree burns are severe burns that affect the tissue layers beneath the skin surface and the tissue beneath that.

Only minor first-degree burns and minor second-degree burns in healthy adults should be self-treated with nonprescription products. If a first-degree burn covers an area larger than 1 percent of the body (approximately the size of the back of your hand), get medical attention. If a second-degree burn covers an area larger than 1 percent of the body, or if it is a deep burn, get medical attention. Any burn on the face or genital region, and burns affecting infants, children, the elderly, diabetics, or someone with a chronic illness should be treated by a doctor.

For minor burns, prompt treatment with cold-water therapy reduces or even eliminates the pain, redness, and swelling. Immediately immerse the burned area in cold, nonrunning water. Keep the burned area in the water until the pain stops—as long as 45 minutes, if necessary. Often cold-water therapy is so effective that no other treatment is necessary. If serious burns are involved, begin cold-water therapy and call for medical help at once.

Most burns are caused by contact with hot objects, but burns can also be caused by electricity and chemicals. Electrical burns may appear minor because most the burn damage is under the skin. Get medical attention for all but the most minor electrical burns. Chemical burns are caused by contact with acid or caustic substances such as lye. These burns can be very serious, especially if they affect the eyes. Carefully remove any clothing that may have the chemical on it and flush the affected area with lots of water for at least 15 minutes. Get medical attention for all but the most minor chemical burns. If the chemical is in the eye, hold the eye open and flush it with tepid water for 15 to 30 minutes. Tilt the head so that the water does not flush chemicals into the other eye. Cover the eye with a clean bandage and get medical help at once.

Sunburn can range from mild to severe. Mild sunburn is red, painful, and feels hot. More severe sunburn is very red and very painful, to the point where clothing or anything else touching the area is intolerable. Fever, chills, and nausea are also symptoms of severe sunburn.

Sunburn can easily be avoided by limiting exposure to the sun by staying indoors or in the shade, wearing protective clothing, and by using a sunscreen product containing PABA, which blocks ultraviolet (UV) light. Infants, children, and the elderly are more susceptible to sunburn; take extra precautions.

Some prescription drugs (including some common antibiotics) can cause photosensitivity, making you have sunburn symptoms even if you have been in sunlight for only a brief period. Ask your doctor if a prescription drug will cause photosensitivity. If it does, be sure to take precautions to avoid exposure to sunlight.

USING BURN AND SUNBURN PRODUCTS

Most burn and sunburn products are formulated for temporary pain relief. Some of these products contain only protectants such as petrolatum (petroleum jelly), allantoin, zinc oxide, glycerin, or cocoa butter. Skin protectants protect the burned area and keep it from drying. Some burn and sunburn products contain anesthetics to temporarily relieve pain. Some anesthetic products also contain antibiotic ingredients that may help prevent secondary infection of the burn. Some products contain only antibiotic ingredients.

All burn and sunburn products are applied directly to the affected area. The most common application forms are creams, ointments, aerosol or pump sprays, and liquids. Cream and ointment products should be applied sparingly using clean fingertips. Rub gently until the product is absorbed; if you can still see the product on the skin after application, you have used too much. Because very little of these products is needed for effective relief, ask your pharmacist to help you select the correct package size to avoid waste. Aerosol and pump sprays should be shaken well before using. Hold the nozzle about 6 inches from the affected area and apply in short bursts of about 1 to 3 seconds.

Burn and sunburn products containing anesthetics should be applied 3 to 4 times daily. The anesthetic affect usually lasts about 15 to 45 minutes.

Your choice of burn and sunburn product will depend on the active ingredients you prefer and the application form that is most convenient for you. Your pharmacist can help you select the brand that is most appropriate for you.

TYPES OF BURN AND SUNBURN PRODUCTS

Anesthetics

The local anesthetics found most commonly in burn and sunburn products are benzocaine, lidocaine, lidocaine hydrochloride, dibucaine, and pramoxine hydrochloride. Some people are sensitive to benzocaine. If a product containing benzocaine seems to make the burned area more painful or redder, stop using it. The amount of anesthetic in a burn product varies from brand to brand. For most effective pain relief, select a brand that contains the highest anesthetic concentration. For benzocaine, the highest available concentration is 20 percent; for lidocaine, 4 percent; for lidocaine hydrochloride, 4 percent; for dibucaine, 1 percent; for pramoxine hydrochloride, 1 percent. Your pharmacist can help you determine the anesthetic concentration of a product.

Other effective anesthetics for burns and sunburn include benzyl alcohol, menthol, and camphor. These anesthetics are usually combined with protectants in a cream or ointment.

Do not use topical anesthetics on severe burns, on minor burns that cover a large area, or on raw or blistered skin.

Topical Hydrocortisone

Topical hydrocortisone is effective for relieving burn pain. These products are very effective for relieving mild sunburn pain. (For more information about hydrocortisone, see the section on topical antibiotics and antiseptics.)

Antibiotics

The most commonly used antibiotic ingredients in burn and sunburn products are quaternary aluminum compounds such as benzalkonium chloride, phenols such as chloroxylenol, and other antibiotics such as povidone-iodine. Antibiotic ingredients in burn products are said to help prevent secondary infection of the burn. However, if signs of infection such as oozing, pus, or increasing redness appear, get medical help. Do not treat an infected burn with nonprescription antibiotics.

SPECIAL CONSIDERATIONS

Children: Consult a doctor about treating all but very minor burns and sunburn in children and infants.

Elderly persons: Consult a doctor about treating all but very minor burns and sunburn in the elderly.

Cautions for Burn and Sunburn Products

Possible side effects: Some people are allergic to benzocaine. If the affected area becomes redder or more painful after applying a product containing benzocaine, stop using the product.

Other medical problems: Consult a doctor about treating any burn if you have diabetes.

Call Your Doctor:

• If you have a severe burn.
• If you have a minor burn that covers a large area.
• If the burn victim is an infant, child, or elderly person.
• If the burn does not get better or gets worse after 7 days.
• If the burn develops symptoms of infection.

BURN AND SUNBURN PRODUCTS AND COMMON BRANDS

TOPICAL ANESTHETICS

Brand Name	Application Form	Anesthetic
After Burn	gel, spray	lidocaine hydrochloride
After Burn Plus	gel, spray	lidocaine hydrochloride
Benzocaine (generic)	cream	benzocaine
Benzocol	cream	benzocaine
Bicozene	cream	benzocaine
Dermoplast	lotion, spray	benzocaine
Dibucaine (generic)	ointment	dibucaine
Kreo-Benz	liquid	benzocaine
Lagol	ointment	benzocaine
Nupercainal	cream, ointment	dibucaine
Phicon	cream	pramoxine hydrochloride
Pontocaine	cream, ointment	tetracaine hydrochloride
Pramagel	gel	pramoxine hydrochloride
Prax	cream, lotion	pramoxine hydrochloride
Soft 'N Soothe	cream	benzocaine
Sting Kill	swab	benzocaine
Tronothane HCl	cream	pramoxine hydrochloride
Xylocaine	ointment	lidocaine

TOPICAL ANESTHETICS WITH ANTIBIOTIC

Brand Name	Application Form	Anesthetic
aeroCaine	spray	benzocaine
aeroTherm	spray	benzocaine
Americaine	ointment, spray	benzocaine
Bactine First Aid	liquid, spray, pump spray	lidocaine hydrochloride
Burn Ointment	ointment	benzocaine
Burntame	spray	benzocaine
Dermacoat	spray	benzocaine
Foille	ointment, spray	benzocaine
Foille Plus	cream, spray	benzocaine
Foille Medicated First Aid	ointment, spray	benzocaine
Lanacane	spray	benzocaine
Medicone Derma	ointment	benzocaine
Medicone Dressing	cream	benzocaine
Medi-Quik	spray	lidocaine hydrochloride
Mercurochrome II	liquid, spray	lidocaine hydrochloride
San Cura	ointment	benzocaine
Solarcaine	cream, lotion, spray	benzocaine
Sting Relief	lotion	benzocaine
Stypt-aid	spray	benzocaine
Tega Caine	spray	benzocaine
Unguentine	ointment, spray, pump spray	benzocaine
Unguentine Plus	cream	lidocaine hydrochloride
Y-Itch	cream	benzocaine

ANTIBIOTICS		
Brand Name	*Application Form*	*Antibiotic*
Betadine	cream, ointment, spray	povidone-iodine
Mediconet	wipe	benzalkonium chloride
Obtundia	cream, liquid, spray	cresol-camphor
Vaseline First Aid Carbolated Petroleum Jelly	ointment	chloroxylenol

PROTECTANTS	
Brand Name	*Application Form*
A and D	ointment
Balmex	ointment
Caldesene	ointment
Comfortine	ointment
Desitin	ointment
Noxzema	cream
Primaderm	ointment
Vaseline Pure Petroleum Jelly	gel
Zinc Oxide (generic)	ointment, paste

COLDS AND ALLERGIES

When Do You Need a Cold or Allergy Medication?
Cold medications are most often used to help relieve the symptoms of the common cold (also called rhinitis) and mild influenza. Among the symptoms of a cold or the flu are runny nose, stuffed nose, sore throat, cough, fever, and earache. Other common symptoms include red, itchy, or watering eyes, sneezing, postnasal drip, and aching muscles. Many nonprescription cold medications combine a decongestant to relieve the symptoms of nasal congestion (stuffed nose) and an antihistamine that may help to reduce the amount of discharge (runny nose). Many other nonprescription cold medications combine a decongestant and an antihistamine with an analgesic to help relieve aching muscles. Nonprescription multisymptom cold medications usually combine a decongestant, an antihistamine, and an analgesic with cough medications. Nasal sprays generally contain only a decongestant.

Allergy medications are used to relieve the symptoms of allergic rhinitis (also sometimes called hay fever or rose fever), including congestion, sneezing, wheezing, sniffles, and red, watery, itchy eyes. Seasonal allergic rhinitis is generally caused by airborne pollen and mold spores and tends to get better or worse depending on the season. Perennial allergic rhinitis is generally caused by house dust, feathers, and animal dander and tends to be present year round. Some nonprescription allergy medications contain only an antihistamine; others contain both a decongestant and an antihistamine.

If you have allergic rhinitis, use a medication designed specifically to relieve only allergy symptoms. Allergy sufferers, particularly those who are allergic to tree pollen, sometimes confuse their allergy symptoms with cold symptoms. People who are allergic to tree pollen often feel the effects most in the spring. If you have cold symptoms in the spring, you may actually be experiencing allergic rhinitis. Discuss your symptoms with your pharmacist if you're not sure. Avoid broad-based cold remedies when treating allergies.

USING COLD AND ALLERGY MEDICATIONS

Nearly everyone gets a cold at least once a year and many people suffer from occasional seasonal rhinitis. Cold and allergy medications are meant for the temporary, short-term relief of the symptoms of the common cold, mild influenza, and mild allergic rhinitis. If you have a cold or the flu, be sure to get extra rest, drink plenty of fluids, and breathe moist air by using a humidifier or vaporizer, in addition to taking a cold medication.

If you have allergic rhinitis, try to avoid the allergen that causes it. For example, if you are one of the 22 million Americans who have hay fever, stay indoors (especially in the morning) when the pollen count is high. Avoid rubbing your eyes. To relieve your symptoms, take an allergy medication containing an antihistamine. For best results, take antihistamines 30 minutes before going outdoors to help keep the symptoms of hay fever from starting.

Many multisymptom cold medications include cough medications. See the section on cough medications for more information about the active ingredients in antitussives and cough suppressants.

In addition to the active ingredients, some cold and allergy medications also contain alcohol, sodium, sorbitol, saccharin, or sucrose. If you should restrict your intake of any of these ingredients, consult your pharmacist about which product is best for you.

Cold and allergy medications usually come as tablets, capsules, liquids, elixirs, or syrups. Your choice of cold medication will depend on the active ingredients you prefer and the form you prefer to take them in. Topical nasal decongestants usually come as sprays or drops. Your pharmacist can help you select the brand that is most appropriate for you.

The symptoms of a common cold or flu usually go away within 7 days, whether or not you take any medication. Stop taking cold medications when your symptoms subside. The symptoms of seasonal allergic rhinitis usually go away when the amount of pollen or mold spores in the air decreases. Stop taking allergy medications when your symptoms subside.

TYPES OF COLD AND ALLERGY MEDICATIONS

Antihistamines

Antihistamines help relieve the runny nose and watery eyes of allergic rhinitis; to a lesser extent, they may help somewhat to relieve the same symptoms of the common cold and flu. The most commonly used antihistamines are brompheniramine maleate, chlorpheniramine maleate, diphenhydramine hydrochloride, doxylamine succinate, phenindamine tartrate, pheniramine maleate, promethazine maleate, pyrilamine maleate, and thonzylamine hydrochloride.

Phenyltoloxamine citrate is found in some cold and allergy medications, but the evidence that this medication is safe and effective is not clear. Phenyltoloxamine medications are not discussed in this book, but your pharmacist can provide information about them.

A major drawback of antihistamines is that they can cause drowsiness. To a degree the sedative effect depends on the individual and the other ingredients in the medication, but in general the drowsiness effect of antihistamines can be ranked as shown in the chart below. Some antihistamine formulations contain caffeine to counteract the sedative effect. Alcohol will increase the sedative effect of antihistamines. Your pharmacist can help you select the brand that is most appropriate for your needs.

If you take a medication containing an antihistamine, use caution when driving, operating heavy machinery, or doing anything else that requires a high degree of mental alertness. Do not drink alcohol.

SEDATIVE EFFECTS OF VARIOUS ANTIHISTAMINES	
Antihistamine	*Sedative Effect*
Diphenhydramine hydrochloride	strong
Doxylamine succinate	strong
Pyrilamine maleate	moderate
Thonzylamine hydrochloride	moderate
Pheniramine maleate	mild
Brompheniramine maleate	mild
Chlorpheniramine maleate	mild

Decongestants
Decongestants help relieve the stuffy nose of the common cold, flu, and allergic rhinitis. The most commonly used nonprescription decongestants are phenylpropanolamine hydrochloride, phenylephrine hydrochloride, and pseudoephedrine hydrochloride.

Topical decongestants (nose sprays) are discussed below.

Combined Decongestants and Antihistamines
Many cold and allergy medications combine an antihistamine with a decongestant to help relieve both stuffy nose and runny nose. It is unclear if the antihistamine ingredient helps much if you have a cold. Antihistamines are most effective for the symptoms of allergies; they have little effect on the symptoms of colds. To a degree, the decongestant ingredient may counteract the sedative effect of the antihistamine. Alcohol will increase the sedative effect of antihistamines. Your pharmacist can help you select the brand that is most appropriate for your needs.

If you take a medication containing an antihistamine, use caution when driving, operating heavy machinery, or doing anything else that requires a high degree of mental alertness. Do not drink alcohol.

Multisymptom Cold Medications
Some multisymptom cold medications combine an antihistamine, a decongestant,

and an analgesic (almost always acetaminophen). It is unclear if the antihistamine ingredient helps much if you have a cold. Other multisymptom formulations include cough medications. The combination of medications used varies from brand to brand. Some formulations are specifically designed to help you sleep. Your pharmacist can help you select the brand that is best for you.

If you take a medication containing an antihistamine, use caution when driving, operating heavy machinery, or doing anything else that requires a high degree of mental alertness. Do not drink alcohol.

Topical Decongestants

Topical decongestants (nose sprays or drops) are a very effective way to relieve the nasal stuffiness of a cold or allergic rhinitis. Most topical decongestants contain either ephedrine, phenylephrine, naphazoline, oxymetazoline, xylometazoline, levodesoxyephedrine or propylhexedrine. Naphazoline may irritate the lining of the nose; discontinue use if this occurs. In general, topical decongestants are not recommended for children under age 6.

The duration of the decongestant effect depends on the active ingredient, as shown in the chart below.

Topical decongestants also contain preservatives, which have no effect on the user. In addition, many topical decongestants also contain various combinations of sorbitol, glycine, camphor, eucalyptol, and menthol. Some topical decongestants also include small amounts of pheniramine maleate, an antihistamine; others may include boric acid and sodium borate. Your pharmacist can help you select the brand that is best for you.

Topical decongestants can become contaminated. Rinse the tip of the container in hot water after use. Don't share the container with others.

Overuse of topical decongestants can lead to a "rebound" effect and actually make the symptoms of nasal congestion worse. Follow the directions on the package and do not use any topical decongestant more often than the label suggests. Stop using topical decongestants when your symptoms subside.

DURATION OF TOPICAL DECONGESTANTS	
Active Ingredient	*Duration of Effect*
Levodesoxyephedrine	2 hours
Propylhexedrine	2 hours
Ephedrine	4 hours
Phenylephrine	4 hours
Naphazoline	6 hours
Oxymetazoline	6 to 8 hours
Xylometazoline	8 to 10 hours

SPECIAL CONSIDERATIONS

Children: Do not give cold or allergy medications to children under 3 years of age except under the advice and supervision of a physician. Follow package directions for children older than 3. Do not give cold medications containing alcohol to children. Cold medications containing aspirin or other salicylates should be avoided in children and adolescents because of the risk of Reye's syndrome. Do not give topical decongestants to children under age 6. Follow package directions for children older than 6.

Pregnant and nursing women: Avoid cold medications containing alcohol if you are pregnant or nursing. Although antihistamines have not been shown to cause harm to unborn children, they should be avoided during pregnancy. Do not take antihistamines if you are nursing. Do not take decongestants if you are pregnant or nursing.

Elderly persons: Do not exceed recommended dose.

Cold and Allergy Medication Abuse

Cold and allergy medications containing alcohol can be abused to produce intoxication. The active ingredients of these medications are not habit-forming.

Cold and Allergy Medication Overdose

Symptoms of antihistamine overdose include convulsions, red face, hallucinations, or coma. Symptoms of decongestant overdose include headache, heart palpitations, vomiting, and slow pulse. Get medical help immediately.

Cautions for Cold and Allergy Medications

Possible side effects: Minor side effects of nonprescription antihistamines include drowsiness, dizziness, dry mouth, intolerance of contact lenses, loss of appetite, and nausea. Discontinue the medication if these side effects become more unpleasant than your cold or allergy symptoms. Serious side effects of antihistamines include rash, change in vision, painful or difficult urination, rapid heartbeat, irritability, fatigue, and nightmares. Call your doctor if any of these serious side effects occur.

Possible drug interactions: Do not take cold or allergy medications containing antihistamines or decongestants if you also take central nervous system depressants, MAO inhibitors, high blood pressure medication, antidepressants, amphetamines, other antihistamines, sedatives, sleeping pills, or tranquilizers.

Other medical problems: If you have high blood pressure, heart disease, diabetes, overactive thyroid, glaucoma, enlarged prostate, kidney disease, asthma, emphysema or other chronic pulmonary disease, or peptic ulcer, check with your doctor before using cold and allergy medications.

Other considerations: See the section on cough medications for additional information about possible side effects, drug interactions, and other possible problems resulting from the use of multisymptom cold medications.

Call Your Doctor:
- If your cold symptoms persist for more than 7 days.
- If your symptoms include high fever, a very sore throat, or breathlessness.
- If a nonprescription cold or allergy medication does not improve your symptoms after 2 to 3 days.
- If your symptoms become worse after 2 to 3 days.
- If you are elderly or weak and think you have influenza.
- If you develop a red rash on your face, trunk, arms, and legs after a few days. You may have measles.

• If you develop a fine red rash along with cold symptoms. You may have rubella (German measles). If you are pregnant and suspect rubella, call your doctor immediately.

COLD AND ALLERGY MEDICATIONS AND COMMON BRANDS

ANTIHISTAMINES
Active ingredient: Brompheneramine

Brand Name	Dose Form
Dimetane	elixir, timed-release tablet

Active ingredient: Chlorpheniramine

Brand Name	Dose Form
Aller-Chlor	tablet, syrup
Chlor-Trimeton	tablet, syrup
Chlor-Trimeton Long-Acting Repetabs	timed-release tablet
Chlor-Trimeton Maximum Strength	tablet
Coricidin	tablet**
Hista-Compound No. 5	tablet**
Pfeiffer's Allergy	tablet
Phenetron Compound	tablet***
Teldrin	timed-release capsule
	** contains acetaminophen
	*** contains aspirin

Active ingredient: Diphenhydramine

Brand Name	Dose Form
AllerMax	caplet
Banophen	capsule, tablet
Benadryl 25	capsule, tablet
Bydramine Cough	syrup
Diphen Cough	syrup
Genahist	elixir
Gen-D-Phen	syrup
Hydramine Cough	syrup
Nidryl	elixir
Nordryl Cough	syrup
Phendry	elixir

Active ingredient: Tripolidine

Brand Name	Dose Form
Actidil	tablet, syrup

DECONGESTANTS

Active ingredient: Phenylephrine

Brand Name	*Dose Form*
Coldonyl	tablet**

Active ingredient: Phenylpropanolamine

Brand Name	*Dose Form*
Bayer Children's Cold	tablet***
Drinophen	capsule*****
Genex	capsule**
Propagest	tablet
St. Joseph Cold Tablets for Children	chewable tablet**

** contains acetaminophen
*** contains aspirin
***** contains acetaminophen and aspirin

Active ingredient: Pseudoephedrine

Brand Name	*Dose Form*
Allerest No Drowsiness	tablet**
Cenafed	syrup, tablet
CoAdvil	caplet****
Dorcol Children's Decongestant	liquid
Dristan Maximum Strength	caplet**
Drixoral Non-Drowsy Formula	extended-release tablet
Excedrin Sinus	caplet, tablet**
Fiogesic	tablet***
Genaphed	tablet
Myfedrine	liquid
Naldegesic	tablet**
Oranyl	tablet
Oranyl Plus	tablet**
Ornex	caplet**
PhenAPAP No. 2	tablet**
Pseudoephedrine (generic)	tablet
Pseudogest	tablet
Sinarest No-Drowsiness	tablet**
Sine-Aid Maximum	caplet**
Sine-Aid Sinus Headache	tablet**
Sine-Off Maximum Strength No Drowsiness Formula	caplet**
Sinutab Maximum Strength Without Drowsiness	tablet**
Sudafed	tablet
Sudafed Children's	liquid
Sudafed Sinus	caplet**
Sudafed 12 Hour	timed-release capsule
Sudanyl	tablet
Super Anahist	tablet**
Tylenol Sinus Maximum Strength	caplet, tablet**
Ursinus Inlay-Tabs	tablet***

** contains acetaminophen
*** contains aspirin
**** contains ibuprofen

ANTIHISTAMINE WITH DECONGESTANT
Active ingredients: Phenylephrine and Brompheniramine

Brand Name	Dose Form
Dexophed (generic)	tablet
Dimetane Decongestant	elixir, tablet

Active ingredients: Phenylephrine and Chlorpheniramine

Brand Name	Dose Form
Alamine	liquid
Dallergy-D	syrup*
Dihistine (generic)	elixir
Dristan Advanced Formula	caplet, tablet**
Dristan AF	tablet**
Histatab Plus	tablet
Novahistine	elixir
Phenhist	elixir
Ru-Tuss	liquid

* alcohol free
** contains acetaminophen

Active ingredients: Phenylpropanolamine and Brompheniramine

Brand Name	Dose Form
Bromatap	elixir
Dimetapp	elixir, tablet
Genatap	elixir

Active ingredients: Phenylpropanolamine and Chlorpheniramine

Brand Name	Dose Form
Alka-Seltzer Plus Cold	tablet***
Allerest	tablet
Allerest Children's	tablet
Allerest Headache Strength	tablet**
Allerest Sinus Pain Formula	tablet**
Allerest 12 Hour	caplet
A.R.M.	caplet
BQ Cold	tablet**
Chlor-Rest	tablet
Chlor-Trimeton Sinus	caplet**
Conex D.A.	tablet
Conex Plus	tablet**
Contac	timed-release capsule
Contac Maximum Strength Cold Formula	caplet
Coricidin D	tablet**
Coricidin Demilets	chewable tablets**
Coricidin Maximum Strength Sinus Headache	tablet**
Covangesic	tablet**
Dehist	capsule
Demazin	syrup

Demazin Repetabs	tablet
Duadacin	capsule**
Extreme Cold Formula	caplet**
4-Way Cold	tablet**
Genamin	syrup*
Gencold	capsule
Myminic	syrup
Myphetapp	elixir
Noraminic	syrup
Pyrroxate	capsule**
Sinapils	tablet**
Sinarest	tablet**
Sinarest Extra Strength	tablet**
Sine-Off Sinus Medicine	tablet***
Sinulin	tablet**
Snaplets-D	granules
Triaminic Allergy	tablet
Triaminic Chewable	tablet
Triaminic Cold	tablet, syrup*
Triaminic-12	timed-release tablet
Triaminicin	tablet**
Trind	liquid
Tri-Nefrin Extra Strength	tablet
Triphenyl	syrup*
Valihist	tablet**

     * alcohol free
     ** contains acetaminophen
     *** contains aspirin

Active ingredients: Phenylpropanolamine and Diphenhydramine

Brand Name	*Dose Form*
Alka-Seltzer Plus Night-Time Cold	tablet***
Benadryl Decongestant Kapseals	capsule
Benadryl Plus	tablet**
Benadryl Plus Nighttime	liquid**
Benylin D	elixir

     ** contains acetaminophen
     *** contains aspirin

Active ingredients: Pseudoephedrine and Brompheniramine

Brand Name	*Dose Form*
Disophrol	tablet
Disophrol Chronotabs	timed-release tablet
Drixoral	timed-release tablet, syrup
Drixoral Plus	timed-release tablet**
Sinutab Allergy Formula Sustained Action	tablet

     ** contains acetaminophen

Active ingredients: Pseudoephedrine and Chlorpheniramine

Brand Name	Dose Form
Chlor-Trimeton Decongestant	tablet
Chlor-Trimeton Long-Lasting Decongestant Repetabs	tablet
Codimal	capsule, tablet**
Comtrex Allergy-Sinus	caplet, tablet**
Co-Pyronil 2 Pulvules	capsule
Dallergy-D	capsule
Dorcol Children's Formula	liquid
Fedahist	tablet
Fedahist Decongestant	syrup
Isoclor	liquid, tablet
Isoclor Timesules	timed-release capsule
Kolephrin	caplet**
Myfedrine Plus	liquid
Napril	tablet
Pedia Care Cold Formula	liquid
PhenAPAP Sinus Headache& Congestion	tablet**
Pseudo-gest Plus	tablet
Ryna	liquid*
Sine-Off Maximum Strength Allergy/Sinus	caplet**
Sinutab Maximum Strength	caplet, tablet**
Singlet	tablet**
Sudafed Plus	tablet, syrup
TheraFlu Flu and Cold Medicine	packet**
Tylenol Allergy Sinus	caplet**

* alcohol free
** contains acetaminophen

Active ingredients: Pseudoephedrine and Tripolidine

Brand Name	Dose Form
Actagen	syrup, tablet
Actifed	syrup, tablet, capsule
Actifed Plus	tablet, capsule**
Actifed 12-Hour	capsule
Allerfrin OTC	syrup, tablet
Aprodine	tablet
Cenafed Plus	tablet
Coryban-D	tablet
Genac	tablet
Triofed (generic)	syrup
Tripodrine	tablet

** contains acetaminophen

MULTISYMPTOM COLD MEDICATIONS
Cough Suppressant (Dextromethorphan) with Decongestant

Brand Name	Dose Form
Bayer Cough Syrup for Children	syrup
Conar	syrup
Halls Mentho-Lyptus Decongestant	liquid
Snaplets-DM	granules
Triaminic-DM	timed-release liquid*
Tricodine Pediatric	liquid
	* alcohol free

COUGH SUPPRESSANT WITH DECONGESTANT AND/OR ANTIHISTAMINE

Brand Name	Dose Form
All-Nite Cold Formula	liquid**
Cerose-DM	liquid
Cheracol Plus	liquid
Co-Apap (generic)	tablet**
Comtrex	tablet, caplet, liquid, liqui-gel**
Congespirin for Children, Aspirin Free	chewable tablet, syrup**
Contac Jr.	liquid**
Contac Nighttime Cold Medicine	liquid**
Contac Severe Cold Formula	caplet**
Dondril Anticough	tablet
Formula 44 Cough Mixture	liquid
Genite	liquid**
Kolephrin/DM	caplet**
Myminicol	liquid*
Nycold Medicine	liquid**
NyQuil Nighttime Cold Medicine	liquid**
Orthoxicol	syrup
Pedia Care Cough-Cold Formula	liquid
Pertussin PM	liquid**
Primatuss Cough Mixture 4	liquid
Quiet Night	liquid
Robitussin Night Relief Colds Formula	liquid**
Snaplets-Multi	granules
TheraFlu Flu, Cold and Cough Medicine	packet**
Threamine DM (generic)	liquid*
Triaminic Nite Light	liquid*
Triaminicol Multi-Symptom Cold	syrup*, tablet
Tricodene Forte	liquid
Trind-DM	liquid
Tussar DM	syrup*
Ty-Cold	tablet**
Tylenol Cold Medication	liquid**
Tylenol Cold No Drowsiness	caplet**
Tylenol Multi-Symptom Cold	caplet, tablet**
Viro-Med	tablet**
	* alcohol free
	** contains acetaminophen

COUGH SUPPRESSANT AND EXPECTORANT (GUAIFENESIN) WITH DECONGESTANT AND/OR ANTIHISTAMINE

Brand Name	Dose Form
Ambenyl-D Decongestant Cough Formula	liquid
Comtrex Cough Formula	liquid**
Conar-A	tablet**
Conar Expectorant	liquid
Conex	liquid
Congestac	caplet
Cough Formula with Expectorant	liquid
Daycare	caplet, liquid**
Dimacol	caplet
Dorcol Children's	syrup
Fedahist Expectorant	liquid
Fedahist Expectorant Pediatric	drops
Fendol	tablet**
Formula 44D Decongestant Cough Mixture	liquid
Formula 44M	liquid**
Myminic Expectorant	liquid
Naldecon DX Adult	liquid*
Naldecon DX Children's	syrup*
Naldecon DX Pediatric	drops
Naldecon EX Pediatric	drops
Noratuss II Expectorant	liquid*
Novahistine DMX	syrup
Poly-Histine Expectorant	syrup
Primatuss Cough Mixture 4D	liquid
Robitussin-CF	syrup
Robitussin-PE	syrup
Ru-Tuss Expectorant	liquid
Sudafed Cough	syrup
Triaminic Expectorant	liquid
Triphenyl Expectorant	liquid
	* alcohol free
	** contains acetaminophen

TOPICAL DECONGESTANTS
Active Ingredient: Levodesoxyephidrine

Brand Name	Application Form
Vicks Inhaler	inhaler

Active Ingredient: Oxymetazoline

Brand Name	Application Form
Afrin 12-Hour	drops, spray
Afrin 12-Hour Cherry	spray
Afrin 12-Hour Menthol	spray

Afrin 12-Hour Pediatric	drops
Allerest	spray
Chlorphed-LA	spray
Coridin	mist
Dristan Long-Lasting	spray
Dristan Long-Lasting Menthol	spray
Duramist Plus	spray
Duration	spray
Duration Mentholated Vapor Spray	spray
4-Way Long Lasting	spray
Genasal	solution
Neo-Synephrine Maximum 12-Hour	pump, spray
Nostrilla Long Acting	spray
NTZ Long Lasting	drops, spray
Sinarest	spray
Sinex-L.A.	spray
Twice-A-Day	solution

Active Ingredient: Phenylephrine

Brand Name	*Application Form*
Alconefrin 12	drops
Alconefrin 25	drops, spray
Alconefrin 50	drops
Doktors	drops, spray
Dristan	spray
Dristan Menthol	spray
4-Way Fast Acting Menthol and Regular	spray
Myci-Spray	spray
Neo-Synephrine Extra	spray, drops
Neo-Synephrine Mild	spray, drops
Neo-Synephrine Pediatric	drops
Neo-Synephrine Regular	drops, jelly, pump, spray
Nostril 1/4% Mild	spray
Nostril 1/2% Regular	spray
Rhinall	drops, spray
Rhinall-10	drops
Sinex	spray
St. Joseph	spray

Active Ingredient: Propylhexedrine

Brand Name	*Application Form*
Benzedrex	inhaler
Dristan	inhaler

Active Ingredient: Xylometazoline

Brand Name	*Application Form*
	drops, spray
Otrivin	drops
Otrivin Pediatric	

COLD AND CANKER SORES

When Do You Need a Cold or Canker Sore Medication?
Cold and canker sore medications are used to relieve the pain and discomfort and help the healing of cold sores (herpes simplex; also called fever blisters), canker sores (aphthous or mouth ulcers), and mouth ulcers from minor injuries. These medications are sometimes also used to relieve teething discomfort in babies.

Cold sores or fever blisters are usually caused by the herpes simplex type 1 virus. These painful and unsightly sores form on the lips and the inside of the mouth. The herpes virus remains dormant in the body even after the cold sore clears up. The sores are called cold sores or fever blisters because infections such as the common cold can cause the sores to recur. Stress, exposure to sun or wind, and hormonal changes such as pregnancy or menstruation can sometimes trigger a recurrence.

Cold sores are very common. They generally heal up without leaving a scar in about 10 to 14 days. In severe cases, antiviral drugs may be prescribed by a physician. In mild cases, ice applied to the sore can help relieve pain. Bland emollient creams such as petroleum jelly or protectants such as Orabase help keep the cold sore moist, which helps prevent secondary infection. Topical local anesthetics in a nondrying base (one without alcohol) can help relieve the discomfort.

Canker sores (aphthous or mouth ulcers) are also very common. Their cause is unknown. Canker sores often occur as a cluster of small yellow spots with red borders on the inside of the bottom lip or inside the cheeks; sometimes they occur on the gum or tongue. Canker sores can also occur as larger craters. In either case, canker sores are very painful and can interfere with normal eating, drinking, and oral health care. Canker sores generally heal up in about 10 to 14 days. Topical local anesthetics such as benzocaine in gel or paste form help relieve discomfort.

Mouth ulcers from minor injuries (traumatic ulcers) such as accidentally biting your tongue or cheek or using a toothbrush too vigorously occur as larger, single ulcers. These ulcers usually heal within a week. Topical local anesthetics such as benzocaine in gel or paste form help relieve discomfort. However, if the ulcer is caused by a broken tooth, orthodontic braces, dentures, or the like, the ulcer will not heal until the cause is removed. Get dental care in these cases.

Teething discomfort in babies can be relieved with topical anesthetics such as benzocaine in gel or paste form. However, the American Dental Association has not accepted any on these products as safe and effective for teething. Discuss teething problems in infants with a doctor.

Although some nonprescription products claim to relieve toothache symptoms, these products have not been accepted by the American Dental Association as safe and effective and are not discussed in this book. Get dental care for toothaches.

USING COLD AND CANKER SORE MEDICATIONS
Most cold sore medications contain a bland emollient cream. Most topical oral anesthetics for canker sores contain an anesthetic, usually benzocaine or

butacaine, in gel, paste, or liquid form. In addition to the anesthetic, many topical oral anesthetics contain alcohol; these should not be used on canker sores. Other topical oral anesthetics contain glycerin or another emollient.

Topical oral anesthetics sometimes also contain saccharin. If you should restrict your intake of any of these ingredients, consult your pharmacist about which product is best for you.

Your choice of cold or canker sore medication will depend on whether you want an anesthetic, whether you want a product containing alcohol, and the most convenient form for applying the product. Your pharmacist can help you select the product that is most appropriate for you.

Cold and canker sore medications are meant to be applied directly to the affected area. Oral protective pastes should be dabbed—not rubbed—onto the problem area to form a thin film. Oral gels should be applied onto the affected area with a clean fingertip or cotton swab to form a thin film. Do not touch the tip of the container to the mouth. Oral liquids often come with an applicator. Be sure to rinse the applicator in hot water before and after using. Avoid eating or drinking for 1 hour after application. Cap containers tightly after use and store them in a cool, dry place.

Topical oral anesthetics are often used to relieve minor denture pain or irritation. Remove the denture, apply the anesthetic and wait for the pain to be relieved. Rinse the mouth well before reinserting the denture. Never use these products under dentures. Serious gum irritation and other problems can result. If your dentures are causing mouth irritation, see your dentist.

TYPES OF COLD AND CANKER SORE MEDICATIONS

Topical Anesthetics

By far the most common anesthetic in topical oral anesthetics is benzocaine. Butacaine is found in some products. Benzocaine and butacaine are both effective for relieving pain and irritation. Some people are allergic to benzocaine. If a canker sore gets worse or more painful after applying a benzocaine product, you may be allergic. Stop using the product.

Aspirin or acetaminophen tablets should never be held against the mouth ulcer or cold sore. This will not relieve the pain and may cause serious tissue damage.

Phenol, Camphor, Menthol, and Other Products

Many emollients and topical oral anesthetics contain small amounts of phenol, camphor, menthol, and eugenol. In small amounts these ingredients are acceptable, although they have not been shown to be safe and effective. In larger amounts or frequent applications, these ingredients can be toxic. When treating cold sores or mouth ulcers avoid products that consist primarily of any of these ingredients.

Hydrogen peroxide and carbamide peroxide should not be used to treat canker sores.

Other Cold Sore Treatments

Numerous folk remedies and herbal treatments are often suggested for cold sores. None have been shown to be effective. Amino acids (L-lysine) and preparations containing *Lactobacillus acidophilus* are considered safe but ineffective. Do not use phenol, silver nitrate, camphor, or hydrocortisone to treat cold sores. Secondary infections of cold sores may be treated with nonprescription topical antibiotic creams containing bacitracin or neomycin. If your cold sores are related to exposure to sun, a lip ointment containing a PABA sunscreen may help prevent recurrence.

SPECIAL CONSIDERATIONS

Infants and children: Use topical oral anesthetics with caution on infants and children. Discuss teething problems with your doctor.

Cold and Canker Sore Medication Cautions

Possible side effects: Increased redness, irritation, or soreness may indicate an allergy to benzocaine. Discontinue.

Call Your Doctor:

• If your cold sore becomes infected.
• If your canker sore does not go away after 2 weeks.
• If your canker sores recur often.

Call Your Dentist:

• If your mouth ulcer is caused by dentures, orthodontic braces, other dental appliances, or a broken tooth.

COLD AND CANKER SORE MEDICATIONS AND COMMON BRANDS

TOPICAL ORAL ANESTHETICS (WITH BENZOCAINE)

Brand Name	Dose Form
Anbesol Gel	gel
Anbesol Liquid	liquid
Anbesol Maximum Strength	liquid, gel
Babee Teething Lotion	liquid
Baby Anbesol Gel	gel
Baby Orajel	gel
Baby Orajel Nighttime Formula	gel
Benzodent	paste
Dalidyne	gel
Foille Plus Spray	spray
Jiffy	liquid
Kank-A Liquid Professional Strength	liquid
Lotion-Jel	gel
Numzident Gel	gel
Numzit Cold Sore Lotion	liquid
Numzit Gel	gel
Numzit Lotion	liquid
Orabase-B with Benzocaine	paste
Orabase-O	paste
Orajel	gel
Orajel CSM	gel

Orajel-D	gel
Orajel Maximum Strength	gel
Orajel Mouth-Aid	gel
Orasept Liquid	liquid
Rid-A-Pain Gel	gel
Tanac Liquid	liquid
Tanac Roll-On	liquid
Tanac Stick	solid

EMOLLIENTS AND PROTECTANTS

Brand Name	Active Ingredients
Amosan	sodium peroxyborate
Blistex Lip Ointment	camphor, phenol, allantoin
Campho-Phenique Gel	phenol, camphor
Campho-Phenique Liquid	phenol, camphor
Cold Sore Lotion	gum benzoin, alcohol
Lip Medex	camphor, phenol
Orabase Plain	pectin, gelatin, mineral oil
Pfeiffer's Cold Sore	gum benzoin, camphor, menthol, alcohol
Tanac	tannic acid

CONTRACEPTIVES

When Do You Need a Contraceptive?

Contraceptives are used to help prevent unwanted pregnancy or to control the number and timing of pregnancies. Condoms cany be used for contraception, but they are primarily used to avoid getting or giving sexually transmitted diseases (STDs) such as gonorrhea or AIDS. This section focuses on vaginal contraceptives (spermicides). Because condoms contain no active ingredients, they are not discussed here.

Vaginal contraceptives are safe, inexpensive, easy to use, and readily available. They are most effective when used consistently and properly.

USING CONTRACEPTIVES

Vaginal contraceptives all contain spermicides. Three spermicides are recognized as being safe and effective for contraception: nonoxynol 9, octoxynol 9, and menfegol. Most vaginal contraceptives today contain nonoxynol 9.

Vaginal contraceptives come in a variety of forms, including foam, cream, jelly, and suppository. Spermicides are most effective when they are used in conjunction with another barrier method of contraception such as a diaphragm, cervical cap, or condom. When spermicides alone are used, foams are probably most effective.

Contraceptive sponges are small, circular polyethylene sponges permeated with nonoxynol 9. The sponge is moistened and inserted into the vagina so as to cover the cervix. Contraceptive sponges combine a spermicide with a barrier.

Spermicides remain effective for anywhere from 2 to 24 hours, depending on the form. Read and follow the package directions carefully for maximum protection. Do not douche for at least 8 hours after intercourse.

Your choice of vaginal contraceptive will depend on the form you prefer. Your pharmacist can help you choose the brand that is most appropriate for you.

TYPES OF VAGINAL CONTRACEPTIVES

Spermicides for Diaphragms and Cervical Caps

Vaginal creams and jellies meant to be used with diaphragms and cervical caps have a lower concentration of spermicide. (Spermicides meant to be used alone may also be used with diaphragms and cervical caps.) To use these products properly, fill the diaphragm or cervical cap one-third full. Position the device over the cervix up to 1 hour before intercourse. Do not remove a diaphragm for at least 6 hours. Add more jelly or cream without removing the diaphragm if intercourse is repeated within 6 hours. After 6 hours, remove the diaphragm, wash it, and add more spermicide if it is inserted again. Cervical caps may be left in position for up to 48 hours. Add more jelly or cream without removing the cervical cap if intercourse is repeated.

Cream and Jelly Spermicides

Vaginal creams and jellies meant to be used alone have a higher concentration of spermicide. These products usually come with an applicator for placing the spermicide into the vagina near the cervix. The spermicide is effective immediately and may be inserted as much as 1 hour before intercourse. Repeat the application if intercourse is repeated. Creams and jellies very occasionally will produce allergic reactions in either partner.

Suppository Spermicides

Vaginal suppositories are placed high in the vagina, where they dissolve. They should be inserted at least 10 to 15 minutes before intercourse. Vaginal suppositories may be stored at room temperature. Always unwrap the suppository before inserting it.

Contraceptive Foams

Contraceptive foams are probably the most effective nonbarrier method. These products usually come with an applicator for placing the spermicide into the vagina near the cervix. The applicator may be filled up to 7 days in advance; prefilled applicators are also available. The spermicide is effective immediately and may be inserted up to 1 hour before intercourse. Repeat the application if intercourse is repeated.

Contraceptive Sponges

Contraceptive sponges have been available since 1983. These small, round sponges contain 1 g of nonoxynol 9. Each sponge is individually packaged.

To use the sponge, wet it thoroughly with clean water and squeeze gently until the sponge is very sudsy. (Do not squeeze the sponge dry. It should remain sudsy.) Insert the sponge so that the concave part covers the cervix. Be careful not to pierce the sponge with a fingernail. Vaginal sponges are effective immediately and remain effective for 24 hours. Intercourse may be repeated without removing the sponge or adding spermicide. The sponge should remain in place for at least 6 hours after the last act of intercourse.

To remove the sponge, insert a finger through the loop on the flat side of the sponge and pull gently and slowly. Contraceptive sponges occasionally break into pieces when removed. If you notice that a piece has broken off the sponge, insert a finger into the vagina and gently remove the piece. Dispose of the sponge in the trash; do not flush it.

Contraceptive sponges should not be used during menstruation or after childbirth, miscarriage, or other termination of pregnancy.

Contraceptive sponges are approximately as effective and safe as a diaphragm. Women who have never had children have fewer accidental pregnancies using contraceptive sponges.

The only vaginal sponges currently available are the Today brand. Whitehall Laboratories, the manufacturer, provides a toll-free help line for women with questions: 1 800 223 2329.

SPECIAL CONSIDERATIONS

Pregnant and nursing women: Ask your doctor about using contraceptives if you are trying to become pregnant, think you may be pregnant, or are nursing.

Contraceptive Cautions

Possible side effects: A small number of people may be sensitive or allergic to spermicides. Symptoms may include burning, irritation, itching, or rash for either partner. Stop using the product if a reaction occurs.

Toxic Shock Syndrome (TSS): Toxic shock syndrome (TSS) is a rare, life-threatening condition that is associated with contraceptive sponge use. It is most common in women under age 30. Symptoms of TSS include the sudden onset of a high fever (over 102°), red rash on the palms and soles, and dizziness due to a sharp drop in blood pressure. Other symptoms include nausea, severe muscle pain, sore throat, irritability, disorientation, and coma. Toxic shock syndrome is potentially fatal. Get medical help immediately.

Other medical problems: Consult your doctor if you are being treated for a sexually transmitted disease. If it is medically important for you to avoid pregnancy, consult your doctor about your choice of contraceptive.

Call Your Doctor:
• If you have symptoms of TSS.
• If you have an allergic reaction to a spermicide.
• If a vaginal sponge is discolored or has a foul smell on removal.
• If your menstrual period is delayed. You may be pregnant.

VAGINAL CONTRACEPTIVES AND COMMON BRANDS

FOAMS WITH NONOXYNOL 9

Brand Name
Because
Delfen
Emko
Emko Pre-Fil
Koromex

JELLIES AND GELS WITH NONOXYNOL 9

Conceptrol
Conceptrol Disposable
Koromex
Ramses
Shur-Seal Gel

SUPPOSITORIES WITH NONOXYNOL 9
Encare
Intercept
Semicid

SPERMICIDES FOR DIAPHRAGMS
Gynol II
Koromex
Koromex Crystal Clear
Ortho-Creme
Ortho-Gynol

CORNS, CALLUSES, AND WARTS

When Do You Need a Corn, Callus, or Wart Product?
Corn, callus, and wart removers are used to treat and remove corns and calluses on the feet and warts on the feet, hands, and other parts of the body.

A corn is a small area of skin, usually on top of a toe, that has thickened and raised up from the skin surface because of constant pressure. The area under the corn is sensitive and becomes painful if pressure is placed on the corn. Sometimes corns form in the web between the fourth and fifth (little) toes. These corns are soft and may be mistaken for athlete's foot. (See the section on athlete's foot for more information.)

Calluses are larger, thickened patches of skin that usually develop on the sides or ball of the foot or on a bunion. As with corns, the area under the callus is sensitive.

In general, corns and calluses are caused by pressure and/or friction—often as a result of footwear that is too tight or fits poorly in some other way. Women who wear high heels may get calluses on the balls of their feet because their shoes increase the pressure there.

Corns and calluses often disappear after several weeks if you wear shoes that fit properly and do not bind. If you have corns or calluses because your foot is not an average size or shape, you may have difficulty finding shoes that fit comfortably. A doctor or podiatrist can advise you about orthotic devices and orthopedic shoes.

Warts (verrucae) are viral infections of the skin and mucous membranes. They are found most frequently in teenagers. Common warts (verruca vulgaris) are generally found on the hands and fingers; they are sometimes found on the face. They are small, raised, hard, white or pink lumps that resemble a tiny cauliflower. Flat warts (verruca plana) generally occur in groups on the face or neck, or the back of the hands or knees. They are small, brown, and smooth. Venereal warts occur near the genitals and anus. Plantar warts (verruca plantaris) occur on the soles of the feet. Because you walk on them, these warts become pushed in and are level with the skin. Often several plantar warts appear next to each other, forming a mosaic pattern on the sole of the foot. Plantar warts are sometimes unnoticeable, but if they become large or occur on the ball or heel of the foot, they may become very annoying.

Only common warts and plantar warts should be treated with nonprescription products. If you have common warts on the face, see your doctor. If you have, or think you have, any other kind of wart, particularly venereal warts, see your doctor. If you are over age 45 and develop warts, see your doctor. You may have a more serious condition such as skin cancer. If you have diabetes or circulatory problems, do not attempt to treat corns, calluses, and warts yourself. See your doctor.

Warts usually go away by themselves within a few months. If the wart is unsightly or uncomfortable, a nonprescription wart remover will often be effective, although the treatment may take a long time.

USING FOOT CARE PRODUCTS

The only drug found to be both safe and effective for the nonprescription treatment of corns, calluses, and warts is salicylic acid. The salicylic acid can be applied to the affected area as a liquid or as a solid disk held in place by a pad. To apply the liquid, first wash and dry the affected area. Apply a drop of the liquid, let it dry, and apply additional drops as needed to cover the area. The liquid forms a flexible film that covers the area. It should be peeled off every 2 to 3 days. For corns and calluses, apply the liquid 1 to 2 times daily for 14 days, or until the corn or callus removed. For warts, apply the liquid 1 to 2 times daily for up to 12 weeks, or until the wart is removed.

The liquid containing the salicylic acid is extremely flammable. Never use it near an open flame. Always seal the container tightly and store it in a cool, dark place. Keep the container away from children.

Solid disks are a somewhat easier way to apply salicylic acid. Select pads that are close to the size of the corn or callus. Place the salicylic disk directly on the affected area and cover it with the pad. Leave the disk in place for no more than 48 hours, then remove it. The soft white skin underneath can be removed by scrubbing gently with a rough towel or pumice stone. Repeat the treatment as needed, but not more than 5 times within a 2-week period.

Your choice of liquid or pad will depend on which method is most convenient for you. Your pharmacist can help you select the brand that is most appropriate for you.

TYPES OF FOOT CARE PRODUCTS

Salicylic Acid

Salicylic acid is the only nonprescription medication that is safe and effective for removing corns, calluses, and warts. Although some people are allergic to salicylic acid when they take it internally as aspirin, the chances of reaction to salicylic acid when used to treat corns, calluses, and warts is very slight.

In some cases salicylic acid can cause the affected area to become red, swollen, or irritated. Occasionally application of the salicylic acid will cause pain in the area. Stop using the product if these side effects occur.

SPECIAL CONSIDERATIONS

Children: Ask your doctor about treating warts in children.

Salicylic Acid Abuse

Salicylic acid in liquid form contains volatile chemicals and smells like airplane glue. These products can be abused by inhaling their vapor.

Salicylic Acid Cautions

Possible side effects: Salicylic acid can irritate normal skin. Avoid getting the liquid form on normal skin. Trim pads to fit the affected area. Stop using the product if redness, swelling, irritation, or pain on application occur.

Other medical problems: Do not treat corns, calluses, or warts yourself if you have diabetes or circulatory problems.

Call Your Doctor:
- If your corns or calluses do not get better or get worse after 14 days of treatment.
- If your wart does not go away after 12 weeks of treatment.
- If you have flat warts or venereal warts.
- If you have diabetes or circulatory problems.
- If you are over age 45 and develop a wart.

CORN, CALLUS, AND WART MEDICATIONS

SALICYLIC ACID PRODUCTS	
Brand Name	*Application Form*
Compound W Wart Remover	liquid, gel
Dr. Scholl's Corn Remover	medicated disks
Dr. Scholl's Liquid Corn Remover	liquid
Dr. Scholl's Wart Remover Kit	liquid
Dr. Scholl's Waterproof Corn Removers	medicated disks
Freezone Corn and Callus Remover	liquid
Gets-It Liquid	liquid
Mosco	ointment
Off Ezy Wart Removal Kit	liquid
Wart-Off	liquid

COUGHS

When Do You Need a Cough Medication?

Cough medications are most often used to help suppress dry coughing with chest congestion and little phlegm (nonproductive coughing) or to help remove phlegm from the upper respiratory area ("wet" or productive coughing), particularly when the cough is a symptom of influenza or the common cold. Many nonprescription cough medications combine an antitussive (cough suppressant) for nonproductive coughing and an expectorant for productive coughing in the same product.

USING COUGH MEDICATIONS

Cough medications are meant for the temporary, short-term relief of coughing due to the common cold or mild influenza. In addition to taking the cough medication, be sure to drink plenty of fluids and breathe moist air by using a humidifier or vaporizer.

Many multisymptom cold medications include an antitussive and an expectorant in combination with decongestants and antihistamines. For more information about these medicines, see the section on cold medications.

In addition to the active ingredients, some cough medications also contain alcohol, sodium, sorbitol, saccharin, or sucrose. If you should restrict your intake of any of these ingredients, consult your pharmacist about which product is best.

Cough medications usually come as liquids or syrups. A few medications come in tablet or other form. Your choice of cough medication will depend on the active ingredients you prefer and the form you prefer to take them in. Your pharmacist can help you select the brand that is most appropriate for you.

The symptoms of a cold or flu usually go away within 7 days, whether or not you take any medication. Stop taking cough medications when your symptoms subside.

TYPES OF COUGH MEDICATIONS

Cough Suppressants

Cough suppressants (antitussives) help relieve the symptoms of dry, nonproductive coughs. They are particularly helpful when the cough interferes with sleeping. Codeine and dextromethorphan are the two most commonlyused antitussives; both offer equally good results. However, because codeine can be abused, the sale of codeine-containing medications is restricted in some states. Codeine should not be used by people with chronic pulmonary disease; in addition, some people are allergic to codeine. For these reasons, few nonprescription cough medications contain codeine. Codeine medications are not discussed in this book, but your pharmacist can provide information about them. Many nonprescription cough suppressant formulas combine dextromethorphan with an expectorant, usually guaifenesin.

Expectorants

Expectorants are usually suggested when you have a productive cough—that is, a "wet" cough that brings up phlegm. The only expectorant that has been shown to be generally safe and effective is guaifenesin. Another cough suppressant, terpin hydrate, is also found in some medications. However, terpin hydrate can cause nausea and vomiting and is not recommended for use in children under age 12. Terpin hydrate medications are not discussed in this book, but your pharmacist can provide information about them.

Many nonprescription expectorant formulas combine guaifenesin with dextromethorphan, a cough suppressant.

SPECIAL CONSIDERATIONS

Children: Do not give cough medications to children under 2 years of age except under the advice and supervision of a physician. Do not give cough medications containing codeine to children under 6 years of age. Do not give cough medications containing alcohol to children. Cough medications containing aspirin or other salicylates should be avoided in children and adolescents because of the risk of Reye's syndrome.

Pregnant and nursing women: No studies have been done to determine the effects on guaifenesin on pregnancy. Dextromethorphan has not been shown to cause problems in pregnancy. Guaifenesin and dextromethorphan have not been shown to cause problems in nursing babies. Avoid cough medications containing codeine or alcohol if you are pregnant or nursing.

Elderly persons: People with chronic pulmonary disease should avoid cough medications containing codeine.

Cough Medication Abuse
Cough medications containing codeine or alcohol can be abused to produce intoxication. Abuse of these medications can lead to dependency. Abuse of cough medications containing dextromethorphan can produce intoxication and bizarre behavior but does not lead to dependency.

Cough Medication Overdose
Cough medications containing guaifenesin only are unlikely to cause problems if an overdose occurs. Symptoms of overdose of cough medications containing dextromethorphan include confusion, drowsiness, dizziness, nausea or severe vomiting, severe nervousness, irritability, and restlessness. Get medical help immediately if an overdose occurs.

Cautions for Cough Medications
Possible side effects: Dextromethorphan or guaifenesin occasionally cause confusion or nervousness; in rare cases these drugs can cause dizziness, drowsiness, nausea or vomiting, or stomach pain. Call your doctor if any of these side effects occur.

Possible drug interactions: Do not take a cough medication containing dextromethorphan if you also take central nervous system depressants or MAO inhibitors.

Other medical problems: If you have smoker's cough, asthma, emphysema, or other chronic pulmonary disease, or if you have glaucoma, high blood pressure, prostate disease, or liver disease, check with your doctor before using cough medications.

Other considerations: Be sure to drink 8 to 10 glasses of liquid a day if you take a cough medication containing guaifenesin.

Call Your Doctor:
• If your cough symptoms persist for more than 7 days.
• If your symptoms include fever, a very sore throat, or breathlessness.
• If your cough is painful.
• If you cough up blood, bloody phlegm, or foul-smelling phlegm.
• If you have a dry cough with no other symptoms.
• If your symptoms do not improve or get worse after 2 to 3 days.
• If you develop a skin rash after using a cough medication containing codeine.

COUGH MEDICATIONS AND COMMON BRANDS

SUPPRESSANTS (DEXTROMETHORPHAN)	
Brand Name	*Dose Form*
Cremacoat I	syrup
Delsym	suspension
DM Cough	syrup
Mediquell	chewy squares
Nycoff	tablet
Pertussin ES	liquid
Pinex	syrup
Pinex Concentrate	syrup

EXPECTORANTS (GUAIFENESIN)

Brand Name	Dose Form
Amonidrin	tablet
Anti-Tuss	syrup
Breonesin	capsule
Colrex Expectorant	liquid
Cremacoat 2	syrup
Genatuss	syrup
GG-Cen	capsule, syrup
Glyate	syrup
Mytussin	syrup
Naldecon Senior EX	liquid*
Nortussin	syrup
Robitussin	syrup
Tussciden Expectorant	liquid
	* alcohol free

SUPPRESSANTS (DEXTROMETHORPHAN) WITH EXPECTORANT (GUAIFENESIN)

Brand Name	Dose Form
Benylin Expectorant	liquid
Cheracol D	syrup
Codistan No. 1	syrup
Genatuss DM	syrup
Guaiatuss DM (generic)	liquid
Halotussin DM (generic)	syrup
Kolephrin GG/DM Expectorant	liquid*
Mytussin DM	syrup
Naldecon Senior DX	liquid*
Pertussin CS	liquid
Phanatuss Cough	syrup
Queltuss	tablet
Robitussin DM	syrup
Silexin	syrup*; tablet
St. Joseph Cough Suppressant for Children	syrup
Tolu-Sed DM	liquid
Vicks Children's Cough	syrup*
	* alcohol free

DANDRUFF AND SEBORRHEA

When Do You Need a Dandruff or Seborrhea Product?
Dandruff products help reduce unsightly white flakes of dead skin (dandruff) on the scalp. Seborrhea products help relieve the scaling and lesions of seborrheic dermatitis.

Dandruff is a common problem, in varying degrees of severity, for about 35 percent of the population. Dandruff is caused when the skin cells of the scalp are naturally replaced by the body at a rapid rate. The dead skin cells on the scalp slough off and appear as white flakes. Why the skin cells turn over so rapidly in some people is unknown. Dandruff is not caused by washing the hair too often. It tends to appear at puberty, get worse in young adults, and level off or even disappear by middle age. Dandruff also tends to be more severe in the late autumn and mildest in the summer months.

Dandruff is a natural part of the body's functioning. It is not a disease and there is no cure. Dandruff can be unsightly and annoying, but it is a very minor medical problem that usually responds well to good hygiene and nonprescription treatments. Simply washing the hair once a day with a mild shampoo often controls dandruff symptoms adequately.

Seborrheic dermatitis (seborrhea) can be considered an extension of dandruff to the scalp, face, and trunk. Symptoms of seborrhea include well-defined yellowish-red lesions along with dry or greasy scales. Seborrhea is sometimes also itchy. If seborrhea-like lesions are found on the elbows, knees, or groin region, or if the lesions are very itchy, you may have psoriasis, dermatitis, or ringworm, not seborrhea. (See the section on dermatitis and psoriasis and the section on athlete's foot and other fungal infections for more information.) The most common form of seborrhea is seborrhea capitis, which affects the scalp, face, and sometimes the outer ear. In newborns, seborrhea capitis is called cradle cap and is quite common. Discuss the treatment of cradle cap with your doctor.

The cause of seborrhea is unknown. Unlike dandruff, seborrhea can get worse when you are under stress. Seborrhea capitis can often be controlled well using nonprescription products similar to those for dandruff. However, seborrhea can sometimes cause infections of the eyelid (blepharitis) and ear infections. Severe cases of seborrhea and infections caused by seborrhea should be treated by a doctor.

USING DANDRUFF AND SEBORRHEA PRODUCTS

Nonprescription dandruff products contain ingredients that either help break up dandruff flakes (keratolytic agents) or that help reduce the rate of cell turnover (cytostatic agents). Some dandruff shampoos are not medicated and contain only detergents. These shampoos are effective because they help break up dandruff flakes and wash them away. When using a nonmedicated dandruff shampoo, massage the scalp vigorously and let the shampoo remain on the scalp for several minutes before rinsing thoroughly.

Some nonprescription dandruff product contain coal tars. Although coal tar products are safe and effective for controlling dandruff, they are unpopular because they are quite odorous and can cause staining of the skin and hair. Coal tar dandruff products are not discussed in this book, but your pharmacist can answer your questions about them.

Seborrhea capitis usually responds well to shampooing with nonprescription dandruff products containing keratolyzing agents. If this treatment is ineffective, nonprescription topical hydrocortisone lotions often help. These lotions should not be used on a regular basis because a "rebound" effect can occur when treatment is stopped. They should never be used to treat dandruff. (For more information about topical hydrocortisone, see the section on dermatitis and psoriasis.)

To use a topical hydrocortisone lotion on the scalp, first shampoo the hair and towel it dry. Apply the lotion directly to the scalp and massage it in.

Dandruff and seborrhea products are available as shampoos, lotions, creams, and ointments. Your choice of product will depend on the active ingredient you prefer and the form you prefer to apply it in. Your pharmacist can help you select the product that is most appropriate for you.

TYPES OF DANDRUFF AND SEBORRHEA PRODUCTS

Cytostatic Agents

Cytostatic agents reduce the turnover time of skin cells on the scalp and thus reduce the amount of visible dandruff flakes. Selenium sulfide and zinc pyrithione are the two most commonly used cytostatic agents. Selenium sulfide is more effective for reducing dandruff flakes. Products containing selenium sulfide must be rinsed very thoroughly from the hair, however, or discoloration may occur. If used frequently, selenium sulfide products may leave an odor on the hair and make the scalp oily.

When using products containing cytostatic agents, be careful not to get them in the eyes or on broken skin. Rinse thoroughly if contact occurs. Selenium sulfide is very toxic if taken internally. Keep containers away from children.

Keratolytic Agents

Keratolytic agents help loosen and break up dandruff flakes and make them easier to wash away. The most commonly used keratolytic agents are sulfur and salicylic acid. These ingredients are safe and effective alone or in combination, but they are not as effective as cytostatic agents for controlling dandruff. Keratolytic agents are most effective when applied as lotions, creams, or ointments.

When using products containing keratolytic agents, be careful not to get them in the eyes, mouth, nose, or on the genitals or broken skin. Rinse thoroughly if contact occurs.

Resorcinol, allantoin, and sodium salicylate are sometimes used as keratolytic agents. The effectiveness of these ingredients has not been proven.

Detergents

Nonmedicated shampoos containing detergents are often helpful for controlling mild cases of dandruff. Common ingredients in detergent shampoos include benzalkonium chloride, benzethonium chloride, isoquinolinium bromides, polyoxyethylene ethers, sodium lauryl sulfate, and triethanolamine, among other ingredients. These shampoos also sometimes contain fragrances and coloring agents.

Antimicrobial Agents

Some dandruff and seborrhea products contain antimicrobial agents such as boric acid, captan, iodoquinol, povidone-iodine, and others. These ingredients are said to help prevent secondary infections. There is no evidence that they do so.

SPECIAL CONSIDERATIONS

Children: Do not treat cradle cap except on the advice of a doctor. Do not treat seborrhea in children under age 2 except on the advice of a doctor.

Call Your Doctor:
• If your seborrhea covers a large area of the skin or scalp.
• If your seborrhea does not improve or gets worse within 2 to 3 weeks.
• If seborrhea occurs in child.
• If you develop a secondary infection of the eyes or ears.

DANDRUFF AND SEBORRHEA PRODUCTS AND COMMON BRANDS

CYTOSTATIC PRODUCTS WITH PYRITHIONE ZINC

Brand Name	*Application Form*
Anti-Dandruff Brylcreem	shampoo
Breck One	shampoo, cream, lotion
Danex	shampoo
DHS Zinc	shampoo
Head & Shoulders	shampoo
Sebex	shampoo
Sebulon	shampoo
Zincon	shampoo
ZNP Bar	bar

CYTOSTATIC PRODUCTS WITH SELENIUM SULFIDE

Brand Name	*Application Form*
Selenium Sulfide (generic)	shampoo, lotion
Selsun Blue	shampoo

KERATOLYTIC PRODUCTS WITH SULFUR

Brand Name	*Application Form*
Rezamid Tinted	lotion
Sulfur-8 Light Hair and Scalp Conditioner	ointment
Sulray	shampoo, cream, soap

KERATOLYTIC PRODUCTS WITH SALICYLIC ACID

Brand Name	*Application Form*
Ionil	shampoo
Ionil Plus	shampoo
Ionil T	shampoo
P&S	shampoo
Sebucare	lotion
SLT Lotion	lotion
Tarlene	lotion
Tarsum	shampoo
X-seb	shampoo
X-seb T	shampoo

KERATOLYTIC PRODUCTS WITH SULFUR AND SALICYLIC ACID

Brand Name	*Application Form*
Diasporal	cream
Fostex Medicated Cleansing	shampoo
Glover's Medicated Ointment	ointment
Meted	shampoo
Meted 2	shampoo
pHisoDan	shampoo
Sebulex Conditioning Shampoo with Protein	shampoo
Sebulex Medicated Shampoo	shampoo
Sebutone	shampoo
Vanseb	shampoo, lotion, cream

DETERGENT SHAMPOOS

Brand Name
Metasep
Ogilvie
Pernox
Scadan
Sulfur-8 Shampoo

DERMATITIS AND PSORIASIS

When Do You Need a Dermatitis or Psoriasis Product?

Dermatitis products help relieve redness, itching, vesicles, weeping, dryness, and swelling of the skin from skin inflammations of various origins. Psoriasis products help relieve the lesions, scaling, and itching of psoriasis.

Dermatitis can have a variety of causes. Contact dermatitis is caused by external contact with an irritant or allergen. Sometimes a strong irritant such as an acid can cause contact dermatitis to appear quickly. More often, irritants such as soap, detergents, cosmetics, and some topical medications cause dermatitis to appear after repeated contact over a long period. A very familiar form of contact dermatitis is "dishpan hands," caused by repeated exposure to detergents, soaps, and water. The symptoms of irritant dermatitis usually appears on the hands, but they can also appear on any part of the body that was in contact with the irritant.

Contact dermatitis is sometimes a reaction to touching something you are allergic to, such as dyes or fragrances in cosmetics, some topical drugs (particularly anesthetics such as benzocaine and lidocaine), nickel, and irritating plants such as poison ivy. (See the section on poison ivy for more information.) Allergic dermatitis usually occurs quickly, generally within 48 hours. The symptoms of allergic dermatitis usually appear on the face and hands, but they can also appear on any part of the body that was in contact with the allergen.

In many cases, contact dermatitis can be avoided by avoiding the irritant or allergen that seems to cause it. For example, wearing cotton-lined vinyl gloves while washing dishes or handling irritating substances or things you are allergic to can help keep dermatitis from recurring.

Dermatitis can be confused with other minor skin ailments such as seborrhea, fungal infections, and psoriasis. (See below for more information about psoriasis; see also the section on dandruff and seborrhea and the section on athlete's foot and other fungal infections.)

Sometimes dermatitis is caused by microorganisms. These cases may require antibiotic treatment under the supervision of a doctor.

Atopic dermatitis is usually found in children and young adults. It is a more severe form of dermatitis that has no known cause. Atopic dermatitis should be treated by a doctor.

Psoriasis is an annoying and unsightly condition that varies greatly in its severity from patient to patient. Psoriasis should be diagnosed and treated by a doctor. Once the diagnosis is made, the doctor may recommend nonprescription products to treat the symptoms. Psoriasis has no cure, but the symptoms can often be helped.

USING DERMATITIS AND PSORIASIS PRODUCTS

Products designed to treat dermatitis fall into 3 categories: astringents, protectants, and topical hydrocortisone.

Astringents are usually applied as soaks or compresses. The affected area can be soaked in an astringent solution, or a compress of washcloths soaked in an astringent solution can be applied to the area, 2 to 4 times daily for 15 to 30 minutes at a time.

Protectants are substances that protect the affected area from further irritation. The protectant should be applied directly to the area as a thin film.

Topical hydrocortisone is used to help relieve itching. These products should be applied 3 to 4 times daily as a thin film that is thoroughly massaged into the skin. (For more information about topical hydrocortisone products see the section on topical antibiotics and antiseptics.)

Dermatitis products are available as creams, lotions, ointments, gels, liquids, and sprays. If the area is weeping and a drying affect is desired, solutions and gels are preferable. If the area is slightly dry, creams and lotions are preferable. If the area is very dry, an ointment is preferable. Sprays, gels, and lotions are easier to use on hairy parts of the body. Your choice of dermatitis product will depend on the active ingredient you prefer and the form you prefer to use it in. Your pharmacist can help you select the brand that is most appropriate for you.

Psoriasis products generally include coal tar, keratolytic agents (substances that help break up dead skin cells and reduce scaling), and/or bland emollients to help relieve dryness and itching. Nonprescription topical hydrocortisone products are sometimes used in severe cases.

Coal tar products are safe and effective but can be unpleasant to use because they are smelly and can stain hair and clothing. Coal tar gels overcome these drawbacks but can dry the skin too much. Coal tar products are also available as creams, ointments, lotions, shampoos, and soaps.

Keratolytic agents help break up psoriasis scales. They are usually applied as creams or ointments 2 to 4 times daily.

Protectants help reduce itching by relieving dry skin. Bland emollients such as white petrolatum or emulsion creams are effective.

TYPES OF DERMATITIS AND PSORIASIS MEDICATIONS

Astringents

Astringents help reduce and dry skin weeping in dermatitis. Two astringent solutions, aluminum acetate (Burow's solution) and witch hazel (hamamelis water) are safe and effective astringents. Aluminum acetate solution or witch hazel should be applied to the affected area as a soak or compress. Aluminum acetate packets and tablets for mixing Burow's solution at home are sold under the brand name Domeboro. Several brands of witch hazel are commonly found in pharmacies. Your pharmacist can help you select the brand that is most appropriate for you.

Zinc oxide is an effective protectant (see below) but its value as an astringent has not been shown. Calamine lotion is effective as an astringent, but may cause crusting. Removing the crusts could cause bleeding and lead to infection.

Protectants

Protectants are creams, ointments, gels, and the like that are spread in a thin layer on areas affected by dermatitis to prevent further irritation. Protectants also help soothe dry skin. Zinc oxide is widely used as a protectant. Calamine lotion, which contains zinc oxide, is also effective. For dry skin, bland protectants such as white petrolatum or cocoa butter are helpful. Other protectants helpful for dry skin in both dermatitis and psoriasis are Aquaphor, Nivea, Albolene, and Lubriderm. Your pharmacist can help you select the brand that is most appropriate for you.

Topical Hydrocortisone

Topical hydrocortisone effectively relieves the itching of dermatitis. Use hydrocortisone only if you are certain the affected area is not infected. These products should always be used very sparingly.

Topical hydrocortisone is sometimes used to relieve the symptoms of psoriasis. The product should be applied sparingly 2 to 4 times a day at the start of a psoriasis outbreak. After that, however, hydrocortisone should be applied only occasionally when symptoms are especially severe. Regular use of topical hydrocortisone on psoriasis can lead to a severe "rebound" effect when you stop using it. If you have psoriasis, discuss the use of topical hydrocortisone with your doctor.

Coal Tar Products

Coal tar has been used effectively for many years to treat psoriasis. Coal tar has an unpleasant odor and can stain hair, skin, bedding, and clothing. Coal tar also makes the skin highly sensitive to sunlight. If you use coal tar, you may become more susceptible to sunburn for at least 24 hours after it is applied. Don't apply coal tar to infected skin. Coal tar products can sometimes make psoriasis worse. If you have psoriasis, discuss the use of coal tar products with your doctor.

Keratolytic Agents

Keratolytic agents help loosen psoriasis scales so that they come off naturally. Salicylic acid, usually in the form of a cream or ointment, is the most commonly used nonprescription keratolytic agent. It is generally combined with coal tar.

Salicylic acid can have serious side effects, including nausea, vomiting, and ringing in the ears, if it is used over too much of the body. Allantoin, resorcinol, and sulfur are other keratolytic agents, although these are not as effective as salicylic acid. If you have psoriasis, discuss the use of salicylic acid and other keratolytic agents with your doctor.

SPECIAL CONSIDERATIONS

Children: Discuss the treatment of dermatitis and psoriasis in children with your doctor.

Cautions for Dermatitis and Psoriasis Products

Possible side effects: Coal tar products can make the skin very sensitive to light and susceptible to sunburn. Protect the skin from sunlight for at least 24 hours after application.

Call Your Doctor:

• If your dermatitis does not improve or gets worse after 7 days of self-treatment.
• If your mild psoriasis does not improve or gets worse after 7 days of self-treatment.
• If you have a severe outbreak of psoriasis.
• If coal tar makes your psoriasis worse.
• If an area affected by dermatitis or psoriasis becomes infected.

DERMATITIS AND PSORIASIS PRODUCTS

COAL TAR PRODUCTS

Brand Name	Application Form
Aquatar	gel
Balnetar	bath oil
Coal Tar Solution (generic)	solution
Denorex	shampoo
Denorex Extra Strength	shampoo
DHS Tar	shampoo
DHS Tar Gel	shampoo
Duplex T	shampoo
Estar	gel
Iocon	shampoo
Ionil T Plus	shampoo
Lavatar	bath oil
L.C.D.	cream
Medotar	ointment
Neutrogena T/Derm	body oil
Neutrogena T/Gel	shampoo, conditioner
Pentrax	shampoo
Psorex	shampoo
Tar-Doak	lotion
Tarpaste	paste
Tegrin	soap
Tersa-Tar	shampoo
Zetar	shampoo

COAL TAR WITH KERATOLYTIC AGENT (SALICYLIC ACID)

Brand Name	Application Form
Ionil T	shampoo
Neutrogena T/Gel Scalp Solution	emollient
Neutrogena T/Sal	shampoo
Oxipor VHC	lotion
Pragmatar	cream
P&S Plus	gel
Tarsum Shampoo/Gel	shampoo
Vanseb-T Cream	shampoo
Vanseb-T Lotion	shampoo

COAL TAR WITH OTHER KERATOLYTIC AGENT

Brand Name	Keratolytic Agent
Alphosyl	allantoin
Kay-San cream	allantoin, resorcinol
Tegrin cream, lotion, shampoo	allantoin

SULFUR

Brand Name	Application Form
Sulfur-8	ointment

DIARRHEA

When Do You Need a Diarrhea Medication?
Diarrhea medications are used to help relieve the symptoms of frequent, loose, watery bowel movements. Diarrhea can have many causes. Often it is caused by a bacterial infection (gastroenteritis and traveler's diarrhea are in this category) or by a virus. Diarrhea from these causes is sometimes called "intestinal flu," "24-hour flu," or "stomach bug." Generally these ailments are minor and self-limiting. They will get better in about 48 hours whether or not you take medication to relieve the symptoms. Be sure to drink plenty of liquids to replace the fluid lost to diarrhea.

Diarrhea can also be caused by food. Overeating, especially of foods that are very spicy, high in fiber, very fatty, or high in sugar, can result in diarrhea. Generally no treatment is necessary. Food allergies, particularly to milk products, can also cause diarrhea. If a particular food gives you diarrhea, the best solution is simply to avoid that food. If you have lactase deficiency (milk allergy), ask your pharmacist about products containing lactase enzymes, such as Lactaid and Lactrase.

Drug-induced diarrhea is quite common. Laxatives and antacids can cause diarrhea and diarrhea is a frequent side effect of antibiotic treatment. If you think your diarrhea is drug-induced, discuss the problem with your pharmacist or physician before taking any nonprescription drug to treat it.

Infection with protozoa can also cause diarrhea. The two most common infectious protozoa are *Giardia lamblia* and *Entamoeba hitolytica.* Hikers, campers, travelers, and people in institutions are most likely to be infected with Giardia. Entamoeba is most likely to infect people in areas with poor sanitation. Both infections can cause severe diarrhea and require medical treatment. If you think your diarrhea is caused by protozoa, see your doctor.

Diarrhea that is persistent or chronic diarrhea (lasting more than 2 weeks) can be caused by many conditions, including diabetes, colitis, and cancer. See your doctor if you have chronic diarrhea.

USING DIARRHEA MEDICATIONS

The only diarrhea medications that are safe and effective contain opiates or opiate-like agents, which help stop intestinal motion, or polycarbophil, which helps to absorb water and solidify the bowel movement. Many diarrhea medications contain adsorbents such as kaolin, pectin, or attapulgite. These medications are safe, but they have not been shown to be effective. Many diarrhea medications also contain a drug, often atropine, scopolamine, or hyoscyamine, to relieve cramping. Nonprescription formulations contain too little of these drugs for them to be effective.

Some diarrhea medications contain bismuth, which is a salicylate related to aspirin. If you are hypersensitive to aspirin, do not use a diarrhea medication containing bismuth. (For more information about aspirin hypersensitivity, see the section on pain relievers.)

In addition to the active ingredients, some diarrhea medications also contain alcohol, pepsin, calcium carbonate, lactose, glycerin, or saccharin. If you should restrict your intake of any of these ingredients, consult your pharmacist about which product is best for you.

Diarrhea medications come as liquids, suspensions, tablets, chewable tablets, and caplets. Your choice of diarrhea medication will depend on the active ingredients you prefer and the form you prefer to take them in. Your pharmacist can help you select the brand that is most appropriate for you.

TYPES OF DIARRHEA MEDICATION

Opiates
Opium, opium powder, or paregoric diarrhea medications work by slowing the action of the intestines. This reduces cramping and allows excess water to be reabsorbed rather than excreted. Opiates are usually effective within 2 to 6 hours. The amount of opium in these medications is quite small and does not have a narcotic effect. However, it is possible for a dependency to develop. In addition, opiates can have a sedative effect that can cause dangerous drug interactions. For this reason, some states restrict the sale of opiate diarrhea medications.

Opiate-Like Medications
Loperamide is a drug that, like opiates, slows the action of the intestines. It is usually effective within 1 to 2 hours. Until recently, loperamide was a prescription drug. It is now available in nonprescription formulations. Loperamide offers all the advantages of an opiate medication with fewer drawbacks.

Polycarbophil

Polycarbophil very effectively absorbs water in the bowel. This reduces the frequency of bowel movements and helps make them more solid. Polycarbophil is taken orally as a chewable tablet.

Adsorbents

Many well-known nonprescription diarrhea medications contain adsorbents such as kaolin, pectin, attapulgite, and bismuth. In general, adsorbents do little to relieve diarrhea, although they are safe to use. Adsorbents are usually in suspension form with added flavoring to make them more palatable. Shake the container well before using. Adsorbents containing bismuth may cause a harmless temporary blackening of the stool. Constipation is a possible side effect.

Adsorbents containing bismuth are effective in preventing and treating traveler's diarrhea.

Anticramping Drugs

Many adsorbent diarrhea medications also contain anticramping agents, usually atropine, scopolamine, and/or hyoscyamine. In prescription doses (such as Lomotil) these drugs can be useful for relieving cramps associated with diarrhea. Nonprescription diarrhea drugs do not contain enough of these drugs for them to have any real effect. In addition, the adsorbent ingredients of the medication may inactivate the anticramping drugs. Anticramping medications are potentially dangerous and should not be used by elderly persons, children under age 6, and anyone with glaucoma.

Lactobacillus Formulations

Much controversy and little information surrounds the use of lactobacillus formulations for the treatment of diarrhea. No studies have documented the effectiveness of these medications for the treatment of diarrhea. They are not discussed in this book, but your pharmacist can provide more information about them.

Oral Rehydration Solutions

The discomfort and inconvenience of diarrhea are less serious than the potential for dehydration from fluid loss. Dehydration can be very dangerous and even life-threatening for infants and children. Oral rehydration solutions help replace the body's lost fluid and lost electrolytes. They should be used only on the advice of a physician. Lytren, Pedialyte, Rehydralyte, and Resol are some common brands.

Adults can easily treat themselves for fluid and electrolyte loss. In one large glass, combine 8 ounces of apple, orange, or other fruit juice with 1/2 teaspoon of honey and a pinch of ordinary table salt. In another large glass, combine 8 ounces of plain or carbonated water and 1/4 teaspoon of baking soda (sodium bicarbonate). Sip from each glass alternately.

SPECIAL CONSIDERATIONS

Children: Diarrhea in children can be serious. If the child is under age 3, call your doctor. Do not give diarrhea medications to children under age 3.

Pregnant and nursing women: Do not use diarrhea medications containing opiates or anticramping ingredients if you are pregnant or nursing. Avoid polycarbophil if you are pregnant.

Elderly persons: Diarrhea in the elderly can be serious. Avoid opiates, adsorbents, and anticramping medications.

Other medical problems: Do not take diarrhea medications containing opiates if you have glaucoma, colitis, or bladder problems. Do take diarrhea medications containing loperamide if you have colitis or diarrhea from antibiotic treatment. Do not take diarrhea medications with anticramping ingredients if you have angina, asthma, chronic bronchitis, glaucoma, hiatus hernia, kidney disease, liver disease, prostate disease, thyroid disease, or ulcers.

Diarrhea Medication Abuse

Diarrhea can be a symptom of laxative abuse, which in turn is a symptom of the pattern of purging behavior known as bulimia.

Diarrhea Medication Overdose

Symptoms of opiate medication overdose include rapid pulse, dizziness, confusion, slurred speech, convulsions, and coma. Get medical help at once. Symptoms of anticramping drug overdose include dilated pupils, rapid pulse, dizziness, hallucinations, fever, agitation, and coma. Get medical help at once. Symptoms of loperamide overdose include constipation, lethargy, and unconsciousness. Get medical advice. The symptom of adsorbent overdose is severe constipation.

Call Your Doctor:
• If you are over age 60 and have other medical problems.
• If a child under age 3 has diarrhea.
• If you are pregnant.
• If you have a chronic medical condition such as diabetes, asthma, heart disease, or peptic ulcer.
• If you pass bloody stools.
• If you have a high fever or abdominal tenderness.
• If you become dehydrated.
• If you lose more than 4 percent of your total body weight from diarrhea.
• If your diarrhea does not go away in 5 to 7 days.

DIARRHEA MEDICATIONS AND COMMON BRANDS

OPIATE WITH ADSORBENT	
Brand Name	*Dose Form*
Amogel PC	suspension*
Corrective Mixture with Paregoric	liquid**
Diabismul	suspension
DIA-quel	liquid**
Donnagel-PG	suspension*,**
Infantol Pink	liquid**
Kaodene with Codeine	suspension
Kaodene with Paregoric	suspension
Parepectolin	suspension
Quiagel PG	suspension*
	* contains anticramping agent(s)
	** contains alcohol

LOPERAMIDE

Brand Name	Dose Form
Immodium A-D	caplet
Immodium A-D	liquid**

** contains alcohol

POLYCARBOPHIL

Brand Name	Dose Form
Equalactin	tablet
FiberCon	tablet
Mitrolan	chewable tablet

BISMUTH

Brand Name	Dose Form
Devrom	chewable tablet
Digestalin	tablet
Pepto-Bismol	chewable tablet, liquid
Percy Medicine	liquid**
Pink Bismuth (generic)	liquid

** contains alcohol

ADSORBENTS

Brand Name	Dose Form
Diar-Aid	tablet
Diarrest	tablet
Diasorb	tablet, liquid
Diatrol	tablet
Donnagel	suspension*,**
Kaodene Non-Narcotic	suspension
Kaolin Pectin Suspension	suspension
Kaopectate	tablet, chewable tablet
Kaopectate Concentrated	suspension
Kao-tin	suspension
K-C	suspension
K-P	suspension
K-Pek	suspension
Quiagel	suspension**
Rheaban	tablet

* contains anticramping agent(s)
** contains alcohol

EAR CARE

When Do You Need an Ear Care Product?

Ear care products are used to relieve the symptoms of minor conditions of the outer ear such as itching, external otitis (inflammation of the skin lining the outer ear canal), "swimmer's ear," and impacted ear wax (cerumen).

Ear problems, even minor ones, can be extremely painful. This can make it difficult to know if self-treatment is appropriate. Do not attempt to treat an ear problem with a nonprescription product if you have severe pain, fever, dizziness, or drainage from the ear, if there is a foreign object in the ear, if your hearing is impaired, if you have a noise or ringing in the ears (tinnitus), or if you think you may have an infection or a perforated eardrum (tympanum). A bruise on the outer ear can lead to painful swelling and "cauliflower ear" (perichondritis). Get medical help if you have any of the above symptoms. Get medical help for any ear problem that involves the middle or inner ear.

Boils on the outer ear are a minor problem that can be very painful. Small boils can be easily treated with compresses of warm tap water applied 3 to 4 times a day for 10 to 15 minutes at a time. This helps open the boil and leads to drainage. An antibiotic ointment can help prevent infection.

USING EAR CARE PRODUCTS

Nonprescription ear care products can contain a variety of ingredients. Products meant to relieve the symptoms of mild external otitis and swimmer's ear generally contain active ingredients that help dry the ear and ear canal and make these areas less hospitable to the bacteria that cause infection. Products meant to soften, loosen, and remove excessive ear wax contain carbamide peroxide.

Ingredients such as antipyrine, benzocaine, and camphor are not considered safe and effective for use in the ear.

Your choice of ear care product will depend on the symptoms you have and the active ingredients you prefer. Your pharmacist can help you select the product that is most appropriate for you.

Ear care products are otic solutions (ear drops) that are meant to be instilled (placed in the outer ear canal). To get the most benefit from these products, it is important to instill the solution properly. Warm the ear drops to body temperature by holding the closed container in your hand or holding it under warm running water for a few minutes. Never heat ear drops. Hot ear drops can damage the ear; heat can damage the ingredients in the drops. Place the drops in the affected ear and tilt the ear up or lie down on the opposite ear for at least 2 minutes. There is no need to place cotton or a cotton swab in the ear. Ear drops can generally be applied as 4 drops in each ear up to 4 times daily.

To use an ear wax softener containing carbamide peroxide, place 5 drops in the affected ear, being careful not to let the applicator tip enter the ear canal. To help the drops remain for at least 15 minutes, tilt the ear up or place a small piece of cotton into the ear canal opening. Flush the ear gently with warm water, using a soft rubber bulb syringe. The treatment can be used twice a day for up to 4 days.

TYPES OF EAR CARE PRODUCTS

Drying Agents

Drying agents are helpful for treating the itchiness and pain of mild external otitis and swimmer's ear. Active ingredients often used in these products include acetic acid (vinegar) or boric acid and/or aluminum acetate combined with water, alcohol, glycerin, and/or propylene glycol.

Acetic acid has been used successfully to treat ear problems for centuries. Boric acid is another old remedy. However, boric acid can be toxic and should be used with caution. Do not use it on children.

Aluminum acetate solution (also known as Burow's solution) is an astringent effective for relieving the itching of dermatitis of the external ear when it is applied as a wet compress. It has a drying effect when placed in the ear canal as drops. Aluminum acetate to make Burow's solution at home are sold under the brand name Domeboro.

Glycerin and propylene glycol are usually used as vehicles for the active ingredients in ear care products. By itself glycerin is considered safe as an emollient, but there is little evidence that it is effective. Products containing propylene glycol are more viscous, which helps the active ingredients stay in contact with the ear longer. Some ear care products also contain benzalkonium chloride as a preservative.

Ear Wax Softeners

Healthy ears clean themselves. There is ordinarily no need to remove ear wax either mechanically (with a cotton swab, for example) or by flushing the ears. However, ear wax (cerumen) can sometimes accumulate in the outer ear and need to be removed. Ear wax softeners contain carbamide peroxide. The effervescent effect of the carbamide peroxide helps loosen and remove debris and wax. The wax may then be removed by flushing the ear with warm water. Carbamide peroxide should not be used to treat itching of the ear canal or swimmer's ear. If you wear a hearing aid, your doctor or audiologist can advise you about treating possible ear wax problems.

SPECIAL CONSIDERATIONS

Children: Carbamide peroxide should not be used to treat children under age 12.

Ear Care Products Cautions

Possible side effects: Propylene glycol may cause allergic reactions or dermatitis if used for a long time.

Possible drug interactions: Do not use a nonprescription ear care product if you also use a prescription ear care drug.

Other medical problems: Do not use nonprescription ear care products if you have or think you might have a punctured eardrum (tympanic membrane perforation).

Call Your Doctor:

• If you have diabetes and develop an outer ear problem.
• If you have a fever.
• If you have a discharge from the ear.
• If you have severe pain in the ear.

- If you are dizzy or have vertigo.
- If you have a foreign object in the ear.
- If your hearing is impaired.
- If you have ringing or noise in the ears (tinnitus).
- If your ear condition does not improve or gets worse in 4 or 5 days.

EAR CARE PRODUCTS AND COMMON BRANDS

DRYING AGENTS

Brand Name	Active Ingredients
Aqua-Otic-B	aluminum acetate, boric acid, acetic acid, propylene glycol, benzyl alcohol
Aurinol (generic)	acetic acid, glycerin
Aurocaine 2	boric acid, isopropyl alcohol
Auro-Dri	boric acid, isopropyl alcohol
Benzodyne	acetic acid, glycerin
Dri/Ear Drops	boric acid, isopropyl alcohol
Ear-Dry	boric acid, isopropyl alcohol
Earsol	alcohol, propylene glycol
Halogen Ear Drops	acetic acid, glycerin
Mollifene Ear Drops	glycerin
Swim-Ear	isopropyl alcohol, glycerin

EAR WAX SOFTENERS

Brand Name	Active Ingredients
Aurocaine Ear Drops	carbamide peroxide, glycerin, propylene glycol
Auro Ear Drops	carbamide peroxide
Debrox Drops	carbamide peroxide, glycerin, propylene glycol
Dents Ear Wax Drops	glycerin
E.R.O.	carbamide peroxide, glycerin
Murine Ear Wax Removal System and Ear Drops	carbamide peroxide, alcohol, glycerin
Otix Ear Drops	carbamide peroxide, glycerin

EYE CARE

When Do You Need an Eye Care Product?
Eye care products are used to relieve the symptoms of minor eye irritations such as itching, stinging, tearing, dryness, and redness. Common causes of minor eye irritation include air pollution, smoke, dust, colds, hay fever and other allergies, contact lenses, wind, sunlight, eye strain, poor lighting, and chlorinated water. In some cases, nonprescription eye care medications may be helpful for relieving the symptoms of conjunctivitis (inflammation of the mucous membrane that lines the inner surface of the eyelids and the surface of the inner eye up to the cornea), blepharitis (inflammation of the eyelid margins), and sty (inflammation of a hair

follicle in the eyelid).

A frequent cause of eye infections such as sties and conjunctivitis is contaminated cosmetics such as eye shadow or mascara. Never share cosmetics. If you feel a cosmetic has caused your eye infection, try using a different brand. Avoid using eye makeup if you have an eye infection.

Minor eye irritations are quite common. They will often clear up quickly by themselves when the source of irritation is removed or when the eyes are rested. If your eye irritation does not get better in 3 or 4 days, call your doctor.

Sties can easily be treated with compresses of warm tap water applied 3 or 4 times a day for 10 to 15 minutes at a time. This helps burst the sty and leads to drainage.

Never use a nonprescription eye care medication if you have blurred vision, eye pain, or something embedded in your eye. Do not use nonprescription eye care medications to treat glaucoma, uveitis, flash burns, corneal ulcers, or tear duct infections. If you have any of these conditions, get medical attention promptly.

USING EYE CARE MEDICATIONS

Nonprescription eye care products fall into 3 categories: artificial tears, decongestants, and eye washes. Artificial tears are used to relieve the burning and itching symptoms of "dry" eyes, conjunctivitis, and minor irritations. Artificial tears are also used sometimes used to moisten hard contact lenses. Decongestants help relieve itching, burning, and redness due to allergies and minor irritations. Eye washes have no active ingredients. They are used to bathe the eyes and flush out pollutants, chlorinated water, irritating particles, and the like.

Artificial tear products usually contain viscosity agents and demulcents. Viscosity agents help wet the eye. Demulcents help protect and lubricate the mucous membranes of the eye and inner eyelid and help relieve dryness and irritation. Most artificial tear formulations also contain a preservative to prevent the growth of microorganisms in the liquid after the sterile container has been opened. The most common preservative is benzalkonium chloride.

Decongestants contain a vasoconstrictor ingredient. Vasoconstrictors make the tiny blood vessels found in the white of the eye contract. This reduces redness caused by allergic conjunctivitis and minor irritation and "whitens" the eye. The most common vasoconstrictor in eye products is phenylephrine. Decongestants often also contain viscosity agents and preservatives. Decongestants sometimes also contain buffering agents to make the formulation have the approximately the same alkalinity as tears. (Tears are slightly alkaline, which is why they taste salty.)

Eye washes contain preservatives, buffers, and tonicity agents. Tonicity agents, like buffers, help make the eye wash have approximately the same alkalinity as tears.

Your choice of eye care product will depend on the active ingredients you prefer. Your pharmacist can help you select the product that is most appropriate for you.

Eye care products are ophthalmic solutions (eye drops) that are meant to be instilled (placed in the eye). To get the most benefit from the medication and to avoid the possibility of infection, it is important to instill the solution correctly. Always wash your hands before instilling drops. Check the container carefully for contamination and dirt. To put in the drops, tilt the head back and up. Pull down gently on the skin below the eye and just above the cheekbone. Place the drops into the pouch of the lower eyelid on the side away from the nose and tear ducts. Close the eyes for a minute or so. Don't rub your eyes after instilling eye medication.

Be sure never to touch the tip of the applicator to the surface of the eye, the eyelid, or anything else. If you do accidently touch the tip, wash it with soap and warm water. Keep the container tightly closed when not in use. Store eye medications is a cool place. Discard any eye care product that is discolored, cloudy, or may have been contaminated.

TYPES OF EYE CARE PRODUCTS

Artificial Tears

Artificial tears contain viscosity agents and preservatives. The most common viscosity agents are cellulose derivatives such as hydroxypropyl methylcellulose. Polyvinyl chloride is used as a combined viscosity and demulcent agent. Polyvinyl chloride may build up on contact lenses and should be avoided if you wear contacts. Methylcellulose tends to be slightly more viscous than polyvinyl chloride and may cause annoying crusts on the eyelids. However, methylcellulose stays in the eye longer than polyvinyl chloride.

Decongestants

Decongestants contain a vasoconstrictor and also usually contain a preservative; decongestants also often contain buffers and viscosity agents. The most common decongestants are phenylephrine hydrochloride, naphazoline hydrochloride, and tetrahydrozoline chloride. These decongestants are very similar to each other. All work by constricting the small blood vessels of the eye and dilating (widening) the pupil. The viscosity agents in decongestant formulations are usually polyvinyl alcohol or hydroxyethylcellulose. (See above for more information about viscosity agents.)

Decongestants help whiten red or bloodshot eyes. They are meant for occasional use only. Overuse of decongestants may cause a rebound effect that can actually make the eye irritation worse. Do not use an eye decongestant if you have glaucoma.

Eye Washes

Eye washes have no active ingredients. They contain both a buffer and a preservative. Boric acid or sodium phosphate are common buffers. Benzalkonium chloride or thimerosal are the most common preservatives.

SPECIAL CONSIDERATIONS

Children: Do not use eye care products on children.

Eye Care Product Abuse

Frequent use of eye care products to relieve red or bloodshot eyes may be an indication of drug or alcohol abuse.

Eye Care Product Cautions
Possible drug interactions: Do not use nonprescription eye care products if you
also use a prescription eye care drug. Although the amount of active ingredients
in nonprescription eye products is very low and will probably cause no interac-
tions, avoid these products if you take antidepressants or an MAO inhibitor.
Other medical problems: Do not use eye care medications if you have glaucoma or
diabetes.
Call Your Doctor:
• If your eye irritation does not get better or gets worse in 3 to 4 days.
• If you have a foreign object embedded in your eye.
• If you have blurred vision.
• If you have eye pain.

EYE MEDICATIONS AND COMMON BRANDS

ARTIFICIAL TEARS

Brand Name	*Viscosity Agent*
Adsorbotear	hydroxyethylcellulose
Akwa Tears	polyvinyl alcohol
Artificial Tears Solution	polyvinyl alcohol
Celluvisc	carboxymethylcellulose
Comfort Tears	hydroxyethylcellulose, polyvinyl alcohol
Hypotears	polyvinyl alcohol
I-Liqui Tears	hydroxyethylcellulose, polyvinyl alcohol
Isopto Alkaline	hydroxypropyl methylcellulose
Isopto Plain	hydroxypropyl methylcellulose
Isopto Tears	hydroxypropyl methylcellulose
Just Tears	hydroxypropyl methylcellulose
Lacril	hydroxypropyl methylcellulose
Liquifilm Forte	polyvinyl alcohol
Liquifilm Tears	polyvinyl alcohol
Milroy Artificial Tears	methylcellulose
Moisture Drops	hydroxypropyl methylcellulose
Murine	polyvinyl alcohol
Muro Tears	hydroxypropyl methylcellulose
Murocel	methylcellulose
Refresh	polyvinyl alcohol
TearGuard	hydroxyethylcellulose
Tearisol	hydroxypropyl methylcellulose
Tears Naturale	hydroxypropyl methylcellulose
Tears Naturale II	hydroxypropyl methylcellulose
Tears Plus	polyvinyl alcohol
Tears Renewed	hydroxypropyl methylcellulose
Ultra Tears	hydroxypropyl methylcellulose

DECONGESTANTS

Brand Name	Vasoconstrictor Agent
AK-Nefrin	phenylephrine hydrochloride
Allerest Eye Drops	naphazoline hydrochloride
Clear Eyes	naphazoline hydrochloride
Collyrium	tetrahydrozoline hydrochloride
Comfort Eye Drops	naphazoline hydrochloride
Degest 2	naphazoline hydrochloride
Eye-Zine	tetrahydrozoline hydrochloride
Isopto-Frin	phenylephrine hydrochloride
Mallazine Drops	tetrahydrozoline hydrochloride
Murine Plus	tetrahydrozoline hydrochloride
Naphcon	naphazoline hydrochloride
Ocu-Phrin	phenylephrine hydrochloride
Optigene III	tetrahydrozoline hydrochloride
Optised	phenylephrine hydrochloride
Phenylzin	phenylephrine hydrochloride
Prefrin Liquifilm	phenylephrine hydrochloride
Relief	phenylephrine hydrochloride
Soothe	tetrahydrozoline hydrochloride
20/20 Eye Drops	naphazoline hydrochloride
VasoClear	naphazoline hydrochloride
VasoClear A	naphazoline hydrochloride
Visine	tetrahydrozoline hydrochloride
Visine A.C.	tetrahydrozoline hydrochloride
Visine Extra	tetrahydrozoline hydrochloride

EYE WASHES

Brand Name	Buffer
Blinx	sodium phosphate
Collyrium Eye Lotion	boric acid, sodium borate
Collyrium for Fresh Eyes	boric acid, sodium borate
Dacriose	sodium phosphate
Eye-Stream	sodium acetate, sodium citrate
Eye Wash	boric acid
Lauro Eye Wash	sodium phosphate
Lavoptik Eye Wash	sodium phosphate, sodium biophosphate
Trisol Eye Wash	sodium phosphate
Zincfrin	phenylephrine hydrochloride

HEMORRHOIDS

When Do You Need a Hemorrhoid Product?
Hemorrhoid products are used to relieve the burning, pain, itching, irritation, swelling, and general discomfort of hemorrhoids (piles). Hemorrhoids are a common and annoying problem among adults, but they are not often serious.

More than half of all adults over age 40 in America have hemorrhoids to some degree. Pregnant women often develop hemorrhoids that clear up soon after delivery. In many cases hemorrhoids are only occasionally troublesome and the symptoms can easily be treated with nonprescription products. However, the symptoms of more serious problems, including fissures, fistulas, inflammatory bowel diseases, and tumors, can be taken for the symptoms of hemorrhoids instead. If you have severe pain, seepage, bleeding, protrusion, prolapse, a lump, or thrombosis in the anorectal area, or if you have a change in your bowel habits, see your doctor promptly.

A common cause of hemorrhoids is straining for a bowel movement. To help avoid straining, eat a diet high in fiber and be sure to drink plenty of liquids. Careful hygiene is also helpful. Cleanse and dry the anorectal area thoroughly after each bowel movement. Avoid scented or colored bathroom tissue. Sitz baths in warm water 2 or 3 times a day for 15 minutes at a time help relieve hemorrhoid symptoms during flare-ups. In more severe cases, your physician may recommend a bulk-forming and/or stool-softening laxative. (See the section on laxatives for more information.)

USING HEMORRHOID PRODUCTS

The active ingredients in hemorrhoid products fall into 4 categories: local anesthetics, vasoconstrictors, protectants, and astringents. Many hemorrhoid products contain more than one active ingredient. Products that contain numerous active ingredients may be less effective because the different ingredients may interfere with each other.

Hemorrhoid products are available as creams, ointments, suppositories, foams, and pads. Cleansing products are available as pads and lotions. Pads are very convenient, particularly when you are away from home.

Ointments, creams, and foams are all equally effective as a way to apply the medication in a hemorrhoid product. Use a finger to apply a thin film of these products to the anal area and the lower anal canal. To apply these products within the rectum, use a finger, the applicator supplied with the product, or a pile pipe. (Your pharmacist can explain the use of applicators and pile pipes to you.)

Suppositories are less effective as an application method and should be avoided, particularly when the patient is confined to bed. If you use a suppository, be sure to unwrap it before insertion. If a rectal suppository becomes too warm, it will soften and be difficult to insert. Store suppositories in a cool place, preferably the refrigerator. Hold softened suppositories under cold running water or place them in the refrigerator to harden them. Do not use a suppository if inserting it causes pain.

Many hemorrhoid products are meant for external use only. Read the label carefully. Do not insert products meant for external use into the rectum.

For best results, apply hemorrhoid products after, not before, bowel movements. Cleanse and dry the anal area thoroughly before applying the product sparingly.

Your choice of hemorrhoid product will depend on the active ingredients you prefer and the form that is most convenient for you. Your pharmacist can help you select the product that is most appropriate for you.

TYPES OF HEMORRHOID MEDICATIONS

Local Anesthetics

Local (topical) anesthetics temporarily help relieve burning, pain, itching, and irritation. These products should be used in the anal region and lower anal canal only.

Benzocaine and pramoxine hydrochloride are the most common local anesthetics considered safe and effective for external use. Benzocaine is most effective as an ointment containing polyethylene glycol. Benzocaine products may be applied up to 6 times daily. Some people develop allergic reactions to benzocaine. If a benzocaine product makes the hemorrhoid symptoms worse, stop using it. Pramoxine hydrochloride is most effective as a cream or jelly. These products may be applied up to 5 times daily. Sensitivity or allergies to pramoxine hydrochloride are rare. A few nonprescription products contain dibucaine or tetracaine as the local anesthetic. These may be applied up to 3 or 4 times daily.

Some nonprescription hemorrhoid products contain local anesthetics such as diperodon hydrochloride, camphor, and phenol. These ingredients have not been shown to be effective.

Vasoconstrictors

Vasoconstrictors cause the small blood vessels in hemorrhoidal tissue to constrict. This relieves itching. Vasoconstrictors do not "shrink" swollen hemorrhoids. They should not be used to control minor bleeding. Vasoconstrictors can have serious side effects and should be avoided whenever possible. In general, do not use a hemorrhoid product containing a vasoconstrictor if you have diabetes, high blood pressure, prostate problems, heart disease, or take an MAO inhibitor.

The most commonly used vasoconstrictors are ephedrine sulfate, epinephrine hydrochloride, and phenylephrine hydrochloride.

Ephedrine sulfate has the most long-lasting effect. The effects are felt within 1 minute and last for 2 to 3 hours. Products containing ephedrine sulfate may be applied up to 4 times daily. Do not use a hemorrhoid product containing ephedrine sulfate if you also take an antidepressant medication or MAO inhibitor.

Epinephrine hydrochloride should be used externally only. The effects are felt quickly and last for 2 to 3 hours. Products containing epinephrine hydrochloride may be applied up to 4 times daily.

The effects of phenylephrine hydrochloride are felt quickly and last for 2 to 3 hours. Products containing phenylephrine hydrochloride may be applied up to 4 times daily.

Protectants

Protectants reduce irritation and itching in the anal area by forming a barrier on the skin. Protectants often also serve as the carrier or base for active ingredients such as local anesthetics or vasoconstrictors. Common protectants considered safe and effective for internal and external use include white petrolatum (petroleum jelly), petrolatum, mineral oil, shark liver oil, cod liver oil, zinc oxide, cocoa butter, and vegetable oil. Of these, the most effective is petrolatum. Glycerin and propylene glycol are safe and effective but should be used externally only. The effectiveness of lanolin has not been proven. In addition, lanolin can sometimes cause allergic reactions.

Astringents

Astringents temporarily help relieve irritation and inflammation in the anal area and help reduce mucus and other secretions. Calamine and zinc oxide are effective astringents for both external and internal use. Witch hazel (hamamelis water), largely because of its alcohol content, is an effective astringent for external use only. Witch hazel is a common ingredient in cleansing pads. Tannic acid should not be used in the anal area.

Antiseptics

Some nonprescription hemorrhoid products contain substances, such as boric acid or resorcinol, that are claimed to be external antiseptics that can help prevent infection. There is no real evidence to show that these products are any more effective than good hygiene with soap and water. Boric acid can be toxic and should be avoided. Resorcinol can be toxic if used in the rectum, although it is considered safe if used externally in the recommended dose.

Other Ingredients

Many hemorrhoid products contain additional ingredients such balsam Peru, live yeast cell derivative, or vitamin E. These ingredients are sometimes claimed to aid healing, although there is no evidence that they do. Various herbal or folk remedies such as burdock, stoneroot, and mullein are sometimes suggested to help relieve hemorrhoid symptoms. There is no evidence that they are effective.

SPECIAL CONSIDERATIONS

Children: Do not treat children with hemorrhoid products.

Pregnant and nursing women: Hemorrhoids are a common problem of pregnancy. Discuss treatment with your doctor.

Elderly persons: Elderly persons who are confined to bed or have limited mobility should avoid suppositories.

Hemorrhoid Product Cautions

Possible side effects: Some people are allergic to benzocaine. If your symptoms get worse after applying a product containing benzocaine, stop using the product.

Possible drug interactions: Do not use a hemorrhoid product containing a vasoconstrictor if you are also taking an antidepressant or MAO inhibitor.

Other medical problems: Do not use a hemorrhoid product containing a vasoconstrictor if you have diabetes, high blood pressure, heart disease, or prostate problems. Do not use any hemorrhoid product if you are being treated for colon or rectal disease.

Call Your Doctor:
• If you have rectal or anal bleeding.
• If you have seepage of mucus or fecal matter.
• If you have a lump or protrusion in the anal or rectal area.
• If you have severe or persistent pain.
• If your symptoms do not get better or get worse after 7 days of self-treatment.

HEMORRHOID PRODUCTS AND COMMON BRANDS

CLEANSING PRODUCTS

Brand Name	Product Form
Balneol	lotion
Gentz Wipes	pads
Mediconet	pads
Preparation H Regular	pads
Preparation H Medicated	pads
Tucks	pads

PROTECTANTS

Brand Name	Protectant
Formulation R	shark liver oil
Preparation H	shark liver oil
Vaseline Pure Petroleum Jelly	white petrolatum

ANESTHETICS

Brand Name	Anesthetic
Americaine ointment	benzocaine
BiCozene cream	benzocaine
Fleet Relief Anesthetic ointment	pramoxine hydrochloride
Lanacane cream	benzocaine
Non-Steroid proctoFoam	pramoxine hydrochloride
Nupercainal ointment	dibucaine
Pontocaine ointment, cream	tetracaine
Tronolane cream, suppository	pramoxine hydrochloride

ASTRINGENT (ZINC OXIDE)

Brand Name	Dose Form
Anumed	suppository
Anusol	suppository
Calmol 4	suppository, cream
CPI	suppository
Hemorrin	suppository, ointment
Nupercainal Suppositories	suppository

ANESTHETIC WITH ASTRINGENT (ZINC OXIDE)

Brand Name	Anesthetic
Anocaine Hemorrhoidal suppository	benzocaine
Anusol ointment	pramoxine hydrochloride
Hemet Hemorrhoidal suppository	benzocaine
Hem-Prep suppository	benzocaine
Medicone Rectal ointment	benzocaine

Medicone Rectal suppository	benzocaine
Primaderm-B ointment	benzocaine
Rectagene Medicated ointment	benzocaine

INSECT STINGS AND BITES

When Do You Need an Insect Sting and Bite Product?

Insect sting and bite products are used to relieve the pain, burning, and itching of mosquito bites, bee stings, and the like.

Stinging insects include bees, bumblebees, yellow jackets, wasps, and hornets. These insects have stingers that inject the venom into the skin. Only bees leave the stinger behind and die afterward. Biting insects and arachnids (8-legged creatures) include mosquitoes, fleas, ticks, and chiggers. Some ants, such as fire ants, both bite and sting simultaneously.

Less than 1 percent of the population is dangerously allergic to insect stings, usually from wasps, yellow jackets, and fire ants. If you know you are allergic to stings of this sort, your doctor can prescribe an emergency syringe that contains epinephrine. Severe allergic reactions to insect stings can be dangerous and even life-threatening. The reaction occurs quickly, generally within 15 minutes. Get emergency medical help at once.

Most people who are allergic to insect stings have mild to moderate reactions, including swelling, intense itching, pain, and hives. See your doctor if you have even a mild allergic reaction to an insect sting; you could suddenly develop a more serious reaction. Even if you are not allergic, multiple insect stings should be treated by a doctor.

Ticks can transmit illnesses to humans. Rocky Mountain spotted fever is carried by several tick species. Lyme disease, now the common tick-borne disease in the United States, is carried primarily by the deer tick. Symptoms of Lyme disease can include a red bull's-eye rash around the site of the tick bite, skin rash, fever, fatigue, arthritis-like pain, and headaches. Lyme disease can be difficult to diagnose because not everyone gets the bull's-eye rash or all the other symptoms; in addition, the deer tick is so small that you may not realize one has bitten you. The best approach to tick-borne illness is prevention. Avoid tall grass, wooded areas, and other areas where ticks are found. Wear long-sleeved shirts, long trousers, socks, and closed footwear when in these areas. Check your skin carefully if you have been in a place where ticks are found.

Dogs can also get Lyme disease. If your pet suddenly develops arthritis, severe lameness, fever, lethargy, loss of appetite, or depression, see your veterinarian.

An excellent approach to preventing insect bites is using an insect repellent containing DEET.

A simple way to relieve pain and itching from an insect sting or bite is to apply ice to the area. To help prevent secondary infection, avoid scratching the area.

USING INSECT STING AND BITE PRODUCTS

Insect sting and bite products help relieve pain and itching in different ways, depending on the formulation of the brand. Many products contain a topical anesthetic. Some products contain counterirritants, while other products contain topical antihistamines. Some products also contain an antibiotic to help prevent secondary infection. Topical hydrocortisone is also very effective. (See the section on topical antibiotics and antiseptics for more information on hydrocortisone.)

Insect sting and bite products are available in a variety of forms, including creams, ointments, gels, sprays, and liquids. Your choice of product will depend on the active ingredient you prefer and the application form that is most convenient for you. Your pharmacist can help you select the brand that is most appropriate for you.

TYPES OF INSECT STING AND BITE PRODUCTS

Topical Anesthetics

The topical anesthetic most commonly used in insect sting and bite products is benzocaine. Other anesthetics include lidocaine, dibucaine, and phenol. Some people are sensitive to benzocaine. If a product containing benzocaine seems to make the area more painful or redder, stop using it.

Counterirritants

Some insect sting and bite products contain counterirritants such as camphor or menthol. The sensation of warmth or coldness created by these ingredients blocks the perception of the discomfort from the sting or bite.

Antihistamines

Some insect sting and bite products contain topical antihistamines, usually diphenhydramine or tripelennamine. These products are safe and effective, but should not be used regularly over long periods of time. Do not use these products on infants or young children.

Ammonium Hydroxide

Ammonium hydroxide is said to "neutralize" insect bites and stings. The effectiveness of this ingredient has not been shown.

Insect Repellents

Insect repellent containing DEET are an effective way to avoid insect bites. These products do not repel stinging insects. Traditional insect repellents such as citronella are not as effective as DEET. Do not use insect repellents on children under age 2. Insect repellents will sting if applied to broken skin or mucous membranes. Avoid inhaling these product or getting them in the eyes, nose, or mouth.

SPECIAL CONSIDERATIONS

Children: Do not use products containing topical antihistamines or DEET on children under age 2.

Insect Sting and Bite Products Cautions

Possible side effects: Some people are sensitive to benzocaine.

Other medical problems: Do not use an insect sting or bite product to treat an allergic reaction or multiple stings.

Call Your Doctor:
- If you have an allergic reaction to an insect sting or bite.
- If you are bitten by a poisonous spider such as a black widow or brown recluse.
- If an insect bite or sting becomes infected.
- If you think you may have Lyme disease.

INSECT STING AND BITE PRODUCTS AND COMMON BRANDS

TOPICAL ANESTHETICS

Brand Name	Application Form	Anesthetic
Americaine	ointment, spray	benzocaine
Bactine Antiseptic/Anesthetic First-Aid Spray	spray, pump spray	lidocaine
BiCozene	cream	benzocaine
Chiggerex	ointment	benzocaine
Chiggerex Liquid	liquid	benzocaine
Dermoplast	spray, lotion	benzocaine
Medicone Derma	ointment	benzocaine
Nupercainal	cream, ointment	dibucaine
Rhuli Spray	spray	benzocaine
Rhuli Cream	cream	benzocaine
Skeeter Stik	stick	lidocaine
Solarcaine	cream, lotion, spray	benzocaine
Sting Kill	swab	benzocaine
Sting Relief	lotion	benzocaine

TOPICAL ANTIHISTAMINES

Brand Name	Application Form	Antihistamine
Di-Delamine	gel, spray	diphenhydramine
Sting-Eze	concentrate	diphenhydramine
Surfadil	lotion	diphenhydramine

COUNTERIRRITANTS

Brand Name	Application Form	Counterirritant
Obtundia First Aid Cream	cream	cresol-camphor
Rhuli Gel	gel	menthol, camphor

LAXATIVES

When Do You Need a Laxative?
Laxatives are most often used to relieve constipation, which can be defined as an unusual reduction in the frequency of bowel movements and the difficult passing of hard, dry stools. Symptoms of constipation include dull headache, low back pain, lower abdomen discomfort, and lassitude.

Constipation has many causes. For many people, it is a result of diet with too little fiber or with insufficient fluids. Lack of exercise and failure to respond to the urge to defecate can also contribute to constipation. Pregnant women sometimes become constipated. Some drugs, including certain analgesics, anticholinergics, psychotherapeutic drugs, cough syrups, hypotensives, and diuretics, can cause constipation. Some diseases of the neurological system and of the large bowel can also cause constipation.

If you must prepare for certain diagnostic procedures, such as a colonoscopy, your physician will recommend a laxative. If you are recovering from certain types of surgery or have had a recent heart attack, your physician may recommend a laxative to reduce straining for a bowel movement.

USING LAXATIVES

Laxatives are meant for the occasional relief of simple constipation. They should not be used on a regular basis. Once regularity returns, discontinue the use of the laxative. Castor oil should not be used to treat constipation.

In addition to the active ingredients, some laxatives also contain sodium, potassium, alcohol, sucrose, dextrose, and other ingredients. If you should restrict your intake of any of these ingredients, consult your pharmacist about which product is best for you.

Laxatives come in many forms: liquid, capsule, emulsion, tablet, suppository, granules, syrup, powder, wafers, chewable tablets, and even chewing gum. Your choice of laxative will depend on the active ingredient you prefer and the form that is most convenient for you. Your pharmacist can help you select the brand that is most appropriate for you.

TYPES OF LAXATIVE

Bulk-Forming Laxatives

Physicians generally recommend bulk-forming laxatives because these most naturally resemble the way the body works. Bulk-forming laxatives contain natural or synthetic polysacchrides and cellulose derivatives such as calcium polycarbophil, malt soup, methylcellulose, or psyllium. When ingested, these substances form emollient gels that help the intestinal contents pass through the intestines more easily. Bulk-forming laxatives are available as tablets, capsules, powders, and granules (malt-soup extract is also available as a liquid). These laxatives should be taken with a full glass of fruit juice or other fluid. Results usually occur in 12 to 24 hours, but may take longer for some people.

Emollient and Lubricant Laxatives

Almost all emollient laxatives contain docusate, which helps to soften the fecal mass and make it easier to pass. Emollient laxatives are often recommended for people who should avoid straining for bowel movements, particularly following surgery or a heart attack or when elimination is painful due to hemorrhoids or other physical problems. These laxatives are available as capsules, liquids, and syrups. Results usually occur in 12 to 72 hours.

Lubricant laxatives contain mineral oil, which coats and softens the fecal mass. However, mineral oil can cause serious side effects. Emollient laxatives should be used only for short-term treatment not longer than one week. Emollient laxatives should not be taken in combination with mineral oil.

Stimulant Laxatives

Stimulant laxatives are effective in the treatment of constipation, but they often cause cramping and the passing of excessive amounts of fluid, and they do not help the body return to normal function. Most stimulant laxatives contain bisacodyl, cascara sagrada, phenolphthalein, or senna. Use stimulant laxatives with caution. Do not use these laxatives for more than one week. Stimulant laxatives are available as suppositories, tablets, enemas, chewable tablets, chewing gum, and liquids. Results usually occur in 6 to 12 hours.

Laxatives containing phenolphthalein or senna may harmlessly discolor urine. Phenolphthalein may harmlessly discolor feces in colors ranging from pink to red. The effects of a single dose of phenophthalein can last for up to 3 days.

Stimulant/Emollient Combinations

Numerous laxative combinations of stimulants and emollients are available. The ratio of stimulant to emollient varies from brand to brand. Daily dosage ranges and time for results also vary from brand to brand. Your pharmacist can help you select the brand that is best for you.

Saline Laxatives

Saline laxatives are those that use some form of chemical salt, such as magnesium citrate, magnesium hydroxide, magnesium sulfate, or sodium biphosphate. These laxatives are not meant for treatment of simple constipation. Rather, they are used to evacuate the bowel, particularly in preparation for an endoscopic examination. Use a saline laxative only on the advice of a doctor. Saline laxatives are available as tablets, liquids, and enemas. Results usually occur in 30 minutes to 3 hours.

Glycerin Laxatives

Glycerin, particularly in suppository form, is an effective way to stimulate a bowel movement, particularly for infants and children. Results usually occur in about 30 minutes or less.

SPECIAL CONSIDERATIONS

Children: Stimulant and saline laxatives and enemas should be avoided.

Pregnant and nursing women: Bulk-forming laxatives are preferred during pregnancy and nursing; stimulant laxatives should be avoided.

Elderly persons: For simple constipation, bulk-forming laxatives are preferred. For constipation resulting from prescription medications or disease, consult your physician.

Laxative Abuse

Laxatives can be abused as a form of weight control and as part of the pattern of purging behavior known as bulimia. The serious consequences of laxative abuse include diarrhea, colon disease, and liver disease. Elderly persons can come to depend on laxatives for stimulating bowel movements.

Laxative Overdose

An overdose of bulk-forming laxatives is unlikely to be harmful and has no symptoms. Contact your doctor if a much larger dose than usual is taken. An overdose of docusate may cause appetite loss, nausea, vomiting, and diarrhea. Contact your doctor if symptoms of an overdose appear. An overdose of bisacodyl may cause vomiting. Contact your doctor if a much larger dose than usual is taken. An overdose of cascara may cause vomiting. Contact your doctor if a much larger dose than usual is taken. An overdose of phenolphthalein may cause vomiting. Get medical help immediately if an overdose occurs. An overdose of senna may cause vomiting. Contact your doctor if a much larger dose than usual is taken. An overdose of malt soup may cause wheezing. Contact your doctor if a much larger dose than usual is taken. An overdose of magnesium citrate, magnesium hydrate, or magnesium sulfate may cause vomiting, fainting, weakness, and fluid depletion. Get medical help immediately if an overdose occurs.

Cautions for Laxatives

Possible side effects: Bulk-forming laxatives may cause intestinal blockage, difficulty in breathing, skin rash, or swallowing difficulty. Emollient laxatives may cause skin rash. Stimulant laxatives may cause skin rash, confusion, irregular heartbeat, muscle cramps, fatigue or weakness, and stomach cramping. Saline laxatives may cause confusion, irregular heartbeat, fatigue or weakness, dizziness, muscle cramps, diarrhea, and cramping. Call your doctor if any of these side effects occur.

Possible drug interactions: Psyllium can decrease the effect of medications containing digitalis or salicylates. Docusate, senna, and phenolphthalein can increase the effect of medications containing digitalis. Do not use laxatives containing senna or phenolphthalein if you also take a diuretic or high blood pressure medication. Do not take antacids with a laxative containing phenolphthalein.

Other medical problems: If you have diabetes, kidney disease, rectal bleeding, high blood pressure, or heart disease, check with your doctor before using any laxative.

Other considerations: Avoid taking a laxative within 2 hours of taking another medication.

Call Your Doctor:

• If your bowel habits have changed suddenly and if the change persists for more than 2 weeks.
• If your symptoms include nausea, vomiting, abdominal pain, cramping, or bloating.
• If you have symptoms of appendicitis, intestinal blockage, or inflamed bowel.
• If a nonprescription laxative does not provide relief within 1 week.
• If you have a disease of the gastrointestinal tract.
• If your symptoms return after using a laxative.
• If you develop a skin rash after using a laxative containing phenolphthalein.

LAXATIVES AND COMMON BRANDS

BULK-FORMING LAXATIVES
Calcium Polycarbophil

Brand Name	Dose Form
Equalactin	tablet
Fiberall	tablet

| FiberCon | tablet |
| Mitrolan | chewable tablet |

Malt Soup

Brand Name	Dose Form
Maltsupex	tablet, liquid, powder
Syllamalt	powder

Methylcellulose

Brand Name	Dose Form
Citrucel	powder
Cologel	liquid

Pysllium

Brand Name	Dose Form
Cillium	powder
Effersyllium	powder
Fiberall Natural	powder
Fiberall (various flavors)	powder, wafer
Hydrocil Instant	powder
Innerclean Herbal Laxative	tablet
Konsyl	powder
Konsyl-D	powder
L.A. Formula	powder
Metamucil (various flavors)	powder
Modane Bulk	powder
Modane Versabran	powder
Naturacil	chewable pieces
Perdiem	granules
Perdiem Fiber	granules
Reguloid Natural	powder
Reguloid Orange	powder
Serutan	powder, granules
Siblin	granules
Swiss Kriss	powder, tablet
Syllact	powder
V-Lax	powder

EMOLLIENT LAXATIVES

Docusate

Brand Name	Dose Form
Afko-Lube	capsule, syrup
Colace	capsule, syrup, liquid
DC 240	capsule
Dialose	capsule
Diocto (generic)	syrup, liquid
Diocto-K	capsule
Dioctolose	capsule

Dioeze	capsule
Dio-Sul	capsule
Disonate	capsule, liquid, syrup
Docusate Calcium (generic)	capsule
Docusate Sodium	capsule, syrup
DOK	capsule, liquid
Doss	syrup
Doxinate	capsule, solution
Duosol	capsule
D-S-S	capsule
Genasoft	capsule
Kasof	capsule
Laxinate 100	capsule
Modane Soft	capsule
Pro-Cal-Sof	capsule
Pro-Sof	capsule, syrup
Regulax SS	capsule
Regutol	tablet
Softenex	drops
Sulfalax Calcium	capsule
Surfak	capsule
Therac Plus	enema
Therevac-SB	enema

Mineral Oil

Brand Name	Dose Form
Agoral	emulsion
Agoral Plain	emulsion
Fleet Mineral Oil	enema
Haley's M-O	emulsion
Kondremul	microemulsion
Neo-Cultol	suspension
Zymenol	emulsion

STIMULANT LAXATIVES

Bisacodyl

Brand Name	Dose Form
Bisco-Lax	suppository
Carter's Little Pills	tablet
Dacodyl	tablet, suppository
Dulcolax	tablet, suppository
Fleet Bagenema #1105	enema
Fleet Bisacodyl	tablet, suppository, enema

Cascara Sagrada

Brand Name	Dose Form
Caroid	tablet
Kondremul with Cascara	microemulsion

Milk of Magnesia-Cascara Suspension	suspension
Nature's Remedy	tablet

Phenolphthalein

Brand Name	Dose Form
Alophen	tablet
Colax	tablet
Espotabs	tablet
Evac-Q-Kit	tablet, suppository, liquid
Evac-Q-Kwik	tablet, suppository, liquid
Evac-U-Gen	chewable tablet
Evac-U-Lax	chewable tablet
Ex-Lax	chewable tablet, tablet
Kondremul with Phenolphthalein	microemulsion
Lax-Pills	tablet
Modane	tablet
Modane Mild	tablet
Phenolax	chewable wafer
Prulet	chewable tablet
Unilax	tablet

Senna

Brand Name	Dose Form
Black Draught	tablet, syrup, granules
Dr. Caldwell's Senna Laxative	liquid
Fletcher's Castoria for Children	liquid
Garfields Tea	dried herbs
Genna	tablet
Senexon	tablet
Senna-Gen	tablet
Senokot	tablet, syrup, suppository, granules
Senokot-X-tra	tablet
Senola	tablet

STIMULANT/EMOLLIENT LAXATIVES

Phenolphthalein/Docusate

Brand Name	Dose Form
Colax	tablet
Correctol	tablet
Disolan	capsule
Doxidan	capsule
Ex-Lax Extra Gentle	sugar-coated tablet
Feen-A-Mint	chewing-gum mint, tablet
Feen-A-Mint Pills	tablet
Femilax	tablet
Laxcaps	capsule
Modane Plus	tablet
Phillip's LaxCaps	capsule
Unilax	tablet

Cascara (Casanthranol)/Docusate

Brand Name	Dose Form
Afko-Lube Lax	capsule
Constiban	capsule
Dialose Plus	capsule
Diocto C (generic)	syrup
Diocto-K Plus	capsule
Dioctolose Plus	capsule
Di-Sosul Forte	tablet
Diothron	capsule
Disanthrol	capsule
Disolan Forte	capsule
DSMC Plus	capsule
D-S-S Plus	capsule
Genasoft Plus	capsule
Peri-Colace	capsule, syrup
Peri-Dos	capsule
Pro-Sof Plus	capsule
Regulace	capsule

SALINE LAXATIVES

Magnesium Citrate

Brand Name	Dose Form
Citrate of magnesia (generic)	solution
Citroma	solution
Citro-Nesia	solution

Magnesium Hydroxide

Brand Name	Dose Form
Concentrated Milk of Magnesia	suspension
Haley's M-O	emulsion
Milk of Magnesia (generic)	liquid
Milk of Magnesia USP	suspension
Milk of Magnesia Concentrated	liquid
Phillip's Milk of Magnesia	suspension, tablet

Magnesium Sulfate

Brand Name	Dose Form
Adlerika	liquid
Epsom salt (generic)	granules

Sodium Biphosphate/Sodium Phosphate

Brand Name	Dose Form
Fleet Enema	enema
Fleet Pediatric Enema	enema
Phospho-Soda	liquid
Sodium Phosphates Oral Solution USP	solution

GLYCERIN LAXATIVES
Glycerin
Brand Name	*Dose Form*
Fleet Babylax	liquid
Glycerin USP (generic)	suppository
Sani-Supp	suppository
Therac Plus	enema
Therevac-SB	enema

MENSTRUAL DISCOMFORT

When Do You Need a Menstrual Discomfort Product?

Menstrual discomfort products are used to help relieve the occasional headache, backache, fluid retention, breast tenderness, and abdominal cramping and pain of menstruation. Some products are designed to help relieve the symptoms of premenstrual stress (PMS), which include fluid retention, tender breasts, irritability, and depression.

More than half of all women have occasional mild menstrual discomfort. The intensity varies from woman to woman and from period to period for individual women. A large percentage of women experience occasional PMS starting a few days before menstruation begins.

USING MENSTRUAL DISCOMFORT PRODUCTS

Much routine menstrual discomfort can be reduced with nonprescription pain relievers such as aspirin, ibuprofen, and acetaminophen. If you are hypersensitive to aspirin, do not use a menstrual discomfort product containing aspirin, ibuprofen, or any other salicylate such as potassium salicylate. (See the section on pain relievers for more information.)

Many menstrual discomfort products contain a pain reliever and a diuretic, often pamabrom, for relieving the symptoms of water retention. Caffeine is sometimes included as a diuretic in menstrual discomfort products. If you should restrict your intake of caffeine, consult your pharmacist about which product is best for you. Diuretic herbal extracts such as uva ursi and buchu are found in some products. There is no evidence to show that these extracts are effective and they are not discussed in this book. Your pharmacist can answer your questions about herbal extracts.

Some menstrual discomfort products also contain an antihistamine, usually pyrilamine. Antihistamines are said to help reduce cramping. These drugs are safe, but they have not been shown to be effective.

Menstrual discomfort and PMS can often be relieved by understanding the cause of the symptoms, moderate exercise, good eating habits (including plenty of nonalcoholic fluids), avoiding salt in the diet, and identifying and reducing stress factors where possible. Mild constipation is a common cause of premenstrual and menstrual discomfort. The problem can be avoided by adding fiber to the diet as menstruation nears. (For more information about constipation, see the section on laxatives.)

Menstrual discomfort products come as tablets, caplets, and capsules. Your choice of menstrual discomfort product will depend on the active ingredients you prefer and the form you prefer to take them in. Your pharmacist can help you select the brand that is most appropriate for you.

TYPES OF MENSTRUAL DISCOMFORT PRODUCTS

Pain Relievers

Pain relievers such as aspirin, ibuprofen, and acetaminophen all help relieve headache, backache, and menstrual cramping. Ibuprofen has been shown to be the most effective of these drugs. Aspirin is next in effectiveness and acetaminophen is least effective. Some pain-relieving products are advertised as being formulated specifically for menstrual discomfort. These products contain only ibuprofen and are no different than ordinary formulations of ibuprofen.

Diuretics

Diuretics are used to help eliminate water accumulated in the body during the premenstrual period and during menstruation. Symptoms of water retention include weight gain, swelling (particularly around the ankles), bloating, and a "full" feeling. Only three drugs are safe and effective diuretics in nonprescription products: ammonium chloride, pamabrom, and caffeine. Ammonium chloride is generally safe, but should not be used by anyone with liver or kidney disease. Pamabrom is a weak but effective diuretic. Caffeine is an effective diuretic. However, the stimulant effects of caffeine may cause sleeplessness, particularly if you also drink caffeine-containing beverages such as coffee, tea, and cola.

Other Ingredients

Some menstrual discomfort drugs contain antihistamines such as pyrilamine maleate or phenyltoloxamine citrate. These drugs are said to help relieve cramping. Although these drugs are considered safe, there is no evidence that they are effective.

Feminine Deodorants

Feminine deodorant sprays have no therapeutic value or medicinal properties. They have no hygienic value and are considered cosmetic products by the Food and Drug Administration (FDA). Likewise, "deodorant" tampons have no hygienic value. These tampons must be labeled as "scented." Some women experience irritation or have allergic reactions to the ingredients in these products.

Douche preparations for feminine cleansing also have no therapeutic value or medical properties. Some douches contain boric acid or povidone-iodine. These ingredients should be avoided, especially by pregnant women. Some women experience irritation or have allergic reactions to the ingredients in these products. Douching is not a contraceptive method.

SPECIAL CONSIDERATIONS

Nursing women: Avoid menstrual discomfort medications if you are nursing.

Toxic Shock Syndrome (TSS): Toxic shock syndrome (TSS) is a rare, life-threatening condition that is associated with tampon use during menstruation. It is most common in women under age 30. Symptoms of TSS include the sudden onset of a high fever (over 102°), red rash on the palms and soles, and dizziness due to a sharp drop in blood pressure. Other symptoms include nausea, severe muscle pain, sore throat, irritability, disorientation, and coma. Toxic shock syndrome is potentially fatal. Get medical help immediately.

You are unlikely to get TSS, but you can reduce the risk by not using tampons. If you use tampons, change the tampon 4 to 6 times a day.

Breast self-examination (BSE): Routine, monthly breast self-examination should be practiced by all women. Early detection of breast problems, particularly breast cancer, is crucial for their successful treatment. BSE is simple and quick; it should be performed just after the end of a menstrual period. Ask your doctor to show you how to do a breast self-examination.

Diuretic Abuse

Diuretics are sometimes abused by people with eating disorders, particularly women with anorexia or bulimia. Diuretic abuse can cause serious problems such as dehydration, muscle cramps, weakness, and coma.

Call Your Doctor:
- If your menstrual period is unusually heavy.
- If you have unusually severe abdominal pain or cramps.
- If your menstrual period lasts much longer than usual.
- If you don't have a menstrual period when expected.
- If you have a vaginal discharge along with blood, pus, pain, itching, foul odor.
- If you think you have toxic shock syndrome (TSS).

MENSTRUAL DISCOMFORT PRODUCTS AND COMMON BRANDS

PAIN RELIEVERS

Brand Name	Active Ingredient
Midol 200	ibuprofen
Pamprin-IB	ibuprofen
Trendar	ibuprofen

DIURETICS

Brand Name	Diuretic Ingredients
Aqua-Ban	ammonium chloride and caffeine
Aqua-Ban Plus	ammonium chloride and caffeine
Fluidex with Pamabrom	pamabrom
Odrinil	pamabrom

ACETAMINOPHEN WITH ANTIHISTAMINE

Brand Name	Antihistamine
Menoplex Tablets	phenyltoloxamine
Menstra-Eze	pyrilamine
Midol Maximum Strength	pyrilamine
Midol Regular Strength	pyrilamine

ASPIRIN WITH DIURETIC AND ANTIHISTAMINE

Brand Name	Diuretic	Antihistamine
Midol Caplets	caffeine	cinnamedrine
Midol for Cramps	caffeine	cinnamedrine

ACETAMINOPHEN WITH DIURETIC AND ANTIHISTAMINE

Brand Name	Diuretic	Antihistamine
Midol PMS	pamabrom	pyrilamine
Multi Symptom Menstrual Discomfort Relief Formula	pamabrom	pyrilamine
Pamprin	pamabrom	pyrilamine
Pamprin Extra Strength	pamabrom	pyrilamine
Pamprin Maximum Cramp Relief	pamabrom	pyrilamine
Premsyn PMS	pamabrom	pyrilamine
Sunril	pamabrom	pyrilamine
Synabrom	pamabrom	cinnamedrine

MOTION SICKNESS

When Do You Need a Motion Sickness Medication?
Motion sickness medications, also called antiemetics, are used to prevent and treat nausea and vomiting resulting from car, boat, train, and air travel and the like. Motion sickness medications are not meant to relieve nausea and vomiting from other causes.

USING MOTION SICKNESS MEDICATIONS

The symptoms of motion sickness include paleness, yawning, nausea, and vomiting. Children between the ages of 2 and 12 are particularly likely to suffer from motion sickness, especially during car travel. The problem can often by reduced or eliminated for a child by placing him or her in a car seat or, for an older child, the front passenger seat. This allows the child to look out the front window and often helps prevent motion sickness.

The only safe and effective motion sickness medications all contain antihistamines. (See the section on cold and allergy medications for more information about antihistamines.) These medications are all taken orally as tablets, chewable tablets, or liquids. For best results, take the medication 30 to 60 minutes before travel begins.

A major drawback of antihistamines is that they can cause drowsiness. Alcohol, tranquilizers, and other sedatives can increase the drowsiness. Use caution when driving, operating heavy machinery, or doing anything else that requires a high degree of mental alertness.

Scopolamine administered through a skin patch may be slightly more effective than antihistamines for relieving motion sickness. Scopolamine is presently available only by prescription. If nonprescription motion sickness drugs are ineffective for you, discuss the problem with your doctor.

TYPES OF MOTION SICKNESS MEDICATIONS

Meclizine

Meclizine hydrochloride is an antihistamine that is safe and effective for the relief of motion sickness. An advantage of meclizine is that a single adult dose is effective for 24 hours. However, meclizine should not be given to children under age 12. Meclizine requires a prescription in Canada.

Cyclizine

Cyclizine hydrochloride is an antihistamine that is safe and effective for the relief of motion sickness. Cyclizine is not as long-lasting as meclizine. Adult doses must be repeated every 4 to 6 hours; the dose for children over age 6 must be repeated every 6 to 8 hours. Cyclizine should not be given to children under age 6. Cyclizine requires a prescription in Canada.

Dimenhydrinate

Dimenhydrinate is an antihistamine that is safe and effective for the relief of motion sickness. Adult doses must be repeated every 4 to 6 hours; the dose for children aged 2 to 12 must be repeated every 6 to 8 hours.

SPECIAL CONSIDERATIONS

Children: Do not give to children under age 2. Avoid giving to children under age 12 if possible.

Pregnant and nursing women: Do not take motion sickness medications for the treatment or prevention of morning sickness. Avoid during pregnancy. Do not use if you are nursing.

Elderly persons: Avoid if you have prostate disease.

Motion Sickness Medication Abuse

Antiemetics are sometimes abused by people with eating disorders such as bulimia or anorexia.

Motion Sickness Medication Overdose

Symptoms of an overdose of motion sickness medication include severe drowsiness, confusion, stupor, weak pulse, shallow breathing coma. Get help at once.

Cautions for Motion Sickness Medications

Possible side effects: Drowsiness is common with motion sickness drugs. Do not drive, operate heavy machinery, or do anything that requires a high level of mental alertness. Other possible but not dangerous side effects include dry mouth, nose, and throat, dizziness, headache, nausea, and fast heartbeat.

Possible drug interactions: Do not take motion sickness medications if you take atropine, clozapine, an MAO inhibitor, or any antidepressant, tranquilizer, sedative, pain reliever, or other antihistamine.

Other medical problems: Do not take motion sickness medications if you have asthma, prostate problems, glaucoma, kidney disease, ulcers, or low blood pressure or are allergic to antihistamines.

Call Your Doctor:

• If you develop a rash, hives, jaundice after taking motion sickness medication.
• If your nausea is severe or if you have severe abdominal pain.
• If you vomit blood.
• If your vomiting continues for more than 2 days.

MOTION SICKNESS MEDICATIONS AND COMMON BRANDS

MECLIZINE

Brand Name	*Dose Form*
Bonine	chewable tablet
Dizmiss	chewable tablet
Meclizine HCl (generic)	chewable tablet, tablet

CYCLIZINE

Brand Name	*Dose Form*
Marezine	tablet

DIMENHYDRINATE

Brand Name	*Dose Form*
Calm-X	tablet
Dramamine	chewable tablet, tablet, liquid
Marmine	tablet
Tega-Vert	capsule
Triptone Caplets	caplet

PAIN RELIEVERS

When Do You Need a Pain Reliever?
Pain relievers (also called internal analgesics) are used to help relieve the minor aches and pains of such common ailments as headache, muscle pain, menstrual discomfort, arthritis, bursitis, the common cold, and toothache. (Refer to the sections on colds and allergies, menstrual discomfort, topical antibiotics and antiseptics, insect stings and bites, and burns and sunburn for more information about other types of pain relievers. See the section on sleep aids for pain relievers meant for nighttime use.) Many pain relievers are also useful for reducing swelling and fever.

Nonprescription pain relievers generally contain one of three active ingredients: aspirin (a salicylate), ibuprofen, and acetaminophen.

USING PAIN RELIEVERS

Minor aches and pains are an inevitable part of life. Almost everyone occasionally gets a headache or has a sore muscle. The choice of which type of pain reliever to use depends on the nature of the pain and on your overall health.

In addition to the active ingredients, some pain relievers also contain alcohol, aluminum hydroxide, caffeine, calcium carbonate, dextrose, fructose, lactose, magnesium carbonate, magnesium oxide, saccharin, sodium, sodium bicarbonate, or sugar. If you should restrict your intake of any of these ingredients, consult your pharmacist about which product is best for you.

Pain relievers are available as tablets, chewable tablets, extended-release tablets, caplets, capsules, effervescent tablets, liquids, elixirs, suppositories, granules, and even chewing gum. The brand names of various pain relievers often contain words such as "extra strength," "arthritis strength," "maximum strength," and the like. This usually indicates that the amount of the active ingredient is larger than the amount in the ordinary dose. Generally the ordinary tablet contains 325 mg of active ingredient and the "extra" tablet contain 500 mg. When the active ingredient is aspirin the larger tablet may contain buffering agents; otherwise, there is little difference.

Your choice of pain reliever will depend on the active ingredient you prefer and the form you prefer to take it in. Consult your pharmacist about which active ingredient is best for you and which brand and dosage level is most appropriate for you.

TYPES OF PAIN RELIEVERS

Aspirin

Aspirin is one of the oldest and most widely used nonprescription drugs. First discovered in 1853, it has been available to consumers since 1899. Aspirin helps to relieve pain, reduce swelling, and reduce fever.

Aspirin is generally a very safe and effective medication when taken to relieve occasional minor pain. About 5 percent of all people taking aspirin will have some heartburn or mild nausea. Aspirin can also cause minor gastrointestinal bleeding. For most people, this bleeding is insignificant and unnoticed. However, alcohol can increase the incidence of gastrointestinal irritation and bleeding. Avoid alcohol if you take aspirin. To reduce gastrointestinal discomfort, take aspirin with food or liquids or try buffered or enteric-coated tablets.

Aspirin can cause problems in people with bleeding disorders, peptic ulcers and other gastric disorders, and in those who have had tonsillectomies or tooth extractions. Aspirin should also be avoided by people with gout. Avoid aspirin if you should restrict sodium in your diet.

Some individuals, particularly those with a history of asthma or urticaria (hives), are hypersensitive to aspirin. Symptoms of a reaction to aspirin include shortness of breath, skin rash, hives, swelling, wheezing, and severe asthma attack. Get medical help at once if an aspirin reaction occurs.

Do not attempt to relieve toothache or mouth pain by placing an aspirin tablet against the painful area. This will not help the problem and can lead to gum ulcers and other tissue damage.

Some medical studies have suggested that a low daily dose of aspirin can help reduce the risk of heart attack. If you wish to take aspirin for this reason, consult your physician first.

Do not use any aspirin product if it has a strong vinegar odor. This means that the aspirin has begun to break down.

Ibuprofen

Ibuprofen has been available as a nonprescription medication since 1984. Ibuprofen helps to relieve pain, reduce swelling, and reduce fever. It is particularly effective for postsurgical dental pain and for menstrual discomfort.

Ibuprofen can cause heartburn, nausea, and mild intestinal bleeding. In general, ibuprofen causes fewer gastrointestinal problems than an equivalent dose of aspirin. Even so, ibuprofen should be avoided by people with peptic ulcers and other gastrointestinal conditions. To reduce gastrointestinal discomfort, take ibuprofen with food or liquid.

Ibuprofen can cause bleeding problems, but these are also less severe than an equivalent dose of aspirin.

Some individuals, particularly those with a history of asthma, hives (urticaria), or hypersensitivity to aspirin, are hypersensitive to ibuprofen. Symptoms of a reaction to ibuprofen include high fever, wheezing, severe asthma attack, rash, and hives. Get medical help at once if an ibuprofen reaction occurs.

Acetaminophen

Acetaminophen helps to relieve pain and reduce fever. Acetaminophen is not as effective for pain relief as aspirin or ibuprofen and it does little to reduce swelling. However, acetaminophen is very effective for reducing fever. Because it does not involve the risk of Reye's syndrome, acetaminophen is often suggested for relieving pain and reducing fever for children. Acetaminophen can also be used safely by those taking medication for high blood pressure.

Some nonprescription medications combine aspirin and acetaminophen. Do not use these formulations if you should avoid aspirin.

Prolonged use of acetaminophen can cause anemia and sometimes liver or kidney problems. If your symptoms do not improve after taking acetaminophen for 2 days, call your doctor.

Other Salicylates

Salicylates related to aspirin include choline salicylate, magnesium salicylate, sodium salicylate, and salsalate. Claims that these drugs are as effective as or better than aspirin have not been fully proven. Another related medication, salicylamide, has not been shown to be effective and safe. These medications are not discussed in this book, but your pharmacist can provide information about them.

SPECIAL CONSIDERATIONS

Children: Give children aspirin and acetaminophen for the reduction of fever only on the advice of a physician. Avoid giving any product containing aspirin or ibuprofen to children or adolescents because of the risk of Reye's syndrome. Do not give ibuprofen to children under 15.

Pregnant and nursing women: Pregnant women should not take aspirin, ibuprofen, or acetaminophen. Nursing women should not take aspirin or acetaminophen and should avoid ibuprofen.

Elderly persons: Aspirin is more likely to cause severe gastrointestinal bleeding in people over age 60. Avoid exceeding the recommended dose of acetaminophen.

Pain Reliever Overdose

Because pain relievers are so commonly used, accidental overdoses by children are frequent and can be serious. Symptoms of aspirin overdose include ringing in the ears, nausea, vomiting, dizziness, fever, convulsions, and coma. Symptoms of ibuprofen overdose include confusion, agitation, severe headache, incoherence, convulsions, and coma. Symptoms of acetaminophen overdose include upset stomach, sweating, irritability, diarrhea, convulsions, and coma. Get medical help at once for any overdose.

Household pets sometimes swallow pain relievers. One acetaminophen tablet can kill a cat. Keep containers tightly closed. Find and discard any dropped tablets.

Cautions for Pain Relievers

Possible side effects: Some people are hypersensitive to aspirin and ibuprofen (see above). Symptoms of a reaction to aspirin include shortness of breath, skin rash, hives, swelling, wheezing, and severe asthma attack. Symptoms of a reaction to ibuprofen include high fever, wheezing, severe asthma attack, rash, and hives. Get medical help at once if an aspirin or ibuprofen reaction occurs.

Aspirin often causes mild nausea, heartburn, or ringing in the ears. If your symptoms are more unpleasant than the side effects, continue taking the drug.

Acetaminophen often causes a feeling of lightheadedness. If your symptoms are more unpleasant than the lightheadness, continue taking the drug.

Ibuprofen often causes dizziness, headache, or nausea. If your symptoms are more unpleasant than the side effects, continue taking the drug.

Possible drug interactions: Do not take any nonprescription pain reliever if you also take a prescription nonsteroidal anti-inflammatory drug. Do not take aspirin if you also take an oral anticoagulant, medication for gout or hypoglycemia, medication for high blood pressure (particularly captopril), a prescription anti-inflammatory drug, or any tetracycline antibiotic. Avoid acetaminophen if you also take an oral anticoagulant. Ibuprofen should be used with caution by those taking oral anticoagulants and high blood pressure medication.

Other medical problems: Aspirin should be avoided by people with bleeding disorders, ulcers and other gastric disorders, gout, and by those who have had tonsillectomies or tooth extractions. Acetaminophen should be avoided by people with liver or kidney disease. Ibuprofen should be avoided by people with congestive heart failure, high blood pressure, or kidney disease.

Call Your Doctor:

• If you take acetaminophen and your symptoms do not improve in 2 days.

• If you notice a hearing loss after taking aspirin.

• If you develop muscle cramps, mouth ulcers, or tingling or numbness in the hands or feet after taking ibuprofen.

• If a nonprescription pain reliever does not improve your symptoms or if they get worse after 2 to 3 days.

PAIN RELIEVERS AND COMMON BRANDS

ASPIRIN	
Brand Name	*Dose Form*
Adult Analgesic Pain Reliever	tablet
Alka-Seltzer	effervescent tablet
Alka-Seltzer Extra Strength	effervescent tablet
Alka-Seltzer Flavored	effervescent tablet

Anacin	tablet, caplet
Anacin Maximum Strength	tablet
Arthritis Pain Formula	tablet*
A.S.A. Enseals	tablet
A.S.A. Suppositories	suppository
Ascriptin	tablet*
Ascriptin A/D	tablet*
Ascriptin Extra Strength	tablet*
Aspercin	tablet
Aspergum	chewing gum
Aspermin	tablet
Aspirtab	tablet
Bayer Aspirin	tablet
Bayer Aspirin Maximum	tablet
Bayer Children's Aspirin	chewable tablet
Bayer 8-Hour Timed Release	timed-release tablet
Buffaprin	tablet*
Buffasal	tablet*
Bufferin	tablet*
Bufferin Arthritis Strength	caplet*
Bufferin Extra Strength	tablet*
Buffex	tablet*
Buffinol	tablet*
Cama Arthritis Pain Reliever	tablet*
Dolcin	tablet*
Ecotrin Regular Strength	tablet
Ecotrin Maximum Strength	tablet
Empirin	tablet
Magnaprin	tablet*
Magnaprin Arthritis Strength	tablet*
Measurin Timed Release	timed-release tablet
Momentum	tablet
Norwich Aspirin	tablet
Norwich Extra Strength	tablet
Stanback Powder	granules
Stanback Max Powder	granules
St. Joseph Aspirin	tablet
St. Joseph Low Dose Adult Aspirin	chewable tablet
Verin	tablet
Wesprin Buffered	tablet*
	* buffered

IBUPROFEN

Brand Name	*Dose Form*
Addaprin	tablet
Advil	tablet
Genpril	tablet
Haltran	tablet
Medipren	tablet, caplet

Motrin-IB	tablet
Nuprin	tablet, caplet
Ultraprin	tablet
Valprin	tablet

ACETAMINOPHEN

Brand Name	*Dose Form*
Acephen	suppository
Aceta	tablet, elixir
Acetaminophen Liquid	liquid**
Acetaminophen Uniserts	suppository
Actamin	tablet***
Actamin Super	tablet***
Aminophen	tablet***
Anacin-3 Regular Strength	tablet
Anacin-3 Children's	chewable tablet, liquid**
Anacin-3 Infants' Drops	liquid
Anacin-3 Maximum Strength	tablet
Apacet	chewable tablet
Arthritis Pain Formula, Aspirin-Free	tablet
Aspirin Free Pain Relief	tablet
Bromo Seltzer	granules
Dapa	tablet
Dapa Extra Strength	capsules
Datril Extra Strength	tablet, caplet
Dolanex	liquid
Dorcol Children's Non-Aspirin Fever & Pain Reducer	liquid
Feverall Childrens'	suppository
Feveral Junior Strength	suppository
Genapap Childrens'	chewable tablet
Genapap Childrens' Elixir	elixir**
Genapap Extra Strength	tablet
Genapap Infants' Drops	liquid**
Genebs	tablet
Genebs Extra Strength	tablet
Halenol	tablet
Halenol Childrens'	liquid**
Halenol Extra Strength	tablet
Liquiprin Childrens' Elixir	elixir
Liquiprin Solution	liquid
Meda Cap	caplet
Meda Tab	tablet
Myapap Drops	liquid**
Neopap	suppository
Oraphen-PD	elixir
Pain-Eze +	tablet
Panadol	tablet
Panadol Childrens' Chewable	chewable tablet
Panadol Childrens' Liquid	liquid**

Panadol Infants' Drops	liquid**
Panex	tablet
Panex 500	tablet
Phenaphen	caplet
Snaplets-FR	granules
St. Joseph Aspirin-Free Infant Drops	liquid**
St. Joseph Aspirin-Free Liquid for Children	liquid**
St. Joseph Aspirin-Free Tablets for Children	chewable tablet
Suppap-120	suppository
Suppap-325	suppository
Suppap-650	suppository
Tapanol Extra Strength	tablet
Tempra Chewable Tablets	chewable tablet
Tempra Drops	liquid**
Tempra Syrup	syrup**
Tenol	tablet
Tylenol Childrens'	chewable tablet, liquid,** elixir**
Tylenol Extra Strength	tablet, caplet, gelcap, liquid
Tylenol Junior Strength	tablet
Tylenol Regular Strength	tablet, caplet
Valadol	tablet
Valorin	tablet***
Valorin Super	tablet***
	** alcohol free
	*** sodium free

ASPIRIN AND CAFFEINE

Brand Name	Dose Form
Cope	tablet*
Gensan	tablet
Salabuff	tablet*
	* buffered

ASPIRIN AND ACETAMINOPHEN

Brand Name	Dose Form
Gemnisyn	tablet

ASPIRIN, ACETAMINOPHEN, AND CAFFEINE

Brand Name	Dose Form
Duradyne	tablet
Excedrin Extra Strength	tablet, caplet
Goody's Extra Strength	tablet
Goody's Headache Powder	powder
Neogesic	tablet
Pain Reliever Tablets	tablet

Salatin	capsule
Supac	tablet
Tenol-Plus	tablet
Trigesic	tablet***
Vanquish	caplet*
	* buffered
	*** sodium free

POISON IVY

When Do You Need a Poison Ivy Product?

Poison ivy products treat and relieve the itching, redness, blisters, and oozing or weeping of plant contact allergic dermatitis caused by contact with poison ivy, poison oak, or poison sumac.

Only about half of all people coming into contact with poison ivy, poison oak, or poison sumac will develop plant contact allergic dermatitis. Whether or not you know if you are allergic, learning to recognize and avoid these plants is a good idea. Poison ivy shrubs and vines are widely found throughout the United States and Canada. Poison oak is less widespread but still common throughout the region. Poison sumac is found chiefly in swampy areas of the eastern and southern United States.

An old adage for avoiding poison ivy is "Leaves of three, let it be." Poison ivy plants are vines or shrubs. They have green, lobe-shaped leaves arranged in clusters of three on stalks. In the autumn, small white berries are also present (the berries are an important food for wild birds). Poison oak plants are bushy. The leaves, which have indentations that make them resemble oak leaves, grow in clusters of three. Poison sumac is a woody shrub or small tree. The leaflets grow in pairs along a stalk.

All parts of poison ivy, poison oak, and poison sumac plants, including the leaves, stems, stalks, and any dead or dry parts, contain an oily resin that causes irritation when it comes in contact with the skin—at any season, not just the summer. You don't have to touch the plant directly to develop contact dermatitis—the resin could get on your shoes, for example, and rub off on your hands hours later when you remove the shoes.

If you know you have been in contact with an irritating plant, wash the affected area with soap and water within 15 to 30 minutes. If the hands are involved, be sure to scrub under the fingernails. Washing can often prevent or reduce the severity of the reaction. If you can't wash within 30 minutes, wash when you can.

Clothing, shoes, and anything else that has been in contact with irritating plants should be thoroughly washed; otherwise, they will continue to cause irritation.

The primary symptom of "poison ivy" (plant contact allergic dermatitis) is an itchy, red, streaky rash that appears anywhere from 12 to 48 hours after contact with the plant. In more severe cases, blistering or oozing will be present. The length of time for the rash to develop and its severity will depend on how sensitive you are to the resin. Because different parts of the body may have been exposed to different concentrations of the poisonous resin, the rash may develop days apart on different parts of the body.

Poison ivy rashes usually appear on the face, neck, arms, hands, legs, and feet. Generally the rash disappears within 14 to 21 days. If the rash covers more than 15 percent of the body, or if it is very severe, or if the eyes, mouth, respiratory tract or genitals are involved, get medical help promptly.

USING POISON IVY PRODUCTS

Poison ivy products fall into 4 categories: anesthetics, anti-itching (antipruritic) agents, antiseptics, and astringents. All are applied directly to the affected area 3 to 4 times daily.

Anesthetics help temporarily relieve burning and itching. Anti-itching products generally contain either an antihistamine, a counterirritant, or hydrocortisone. Most poison ivy preparations contain an anesthetic, an anti-itching agent, or both. Antiseptics are found in some poison ivy products. These ingredients are said to help prevent secondary infection, but their value has not been shown and they are not discussed here. Astringents help dry the affected area and promote healing. Many poison ivy products combine 2 or more ingredients.

For severe or widespread cases of poison ivy, colloidal oatmeal baths can be very soothing. Aveeno brand soap, powder, treatment, and lotion contain colloidal oatmeal.

Poison ivy products are available as liquids, lotions, creams, ointments, gels, and sprays. Your choice of poison ivy product will depend on the active ingredient you prefer and the application form that is most convenient for you. Your pharmacist can help you select the brand that is most appropriate for you.

TYPES OF POISON IVY PRODUCTS

Local Anesthetics
Local anesthetics are sometimes helpful for relieving itching and burning from poison ivy. The most commonly used local anesthetics are benzocaine, diperodon, dibucaine, tetracaine, and pramoxine. Some people are sensitive to benzocaine. If your poison ivy rash gets redder or itchier after applying benzocaine, stop using it. Local anesthetics are often combined with anti-itching agents.

Anti-Itching Agents
Several different types of anti-itching (antipruritic) agents are effective for poison ivy. Counterirritant "shake lotions" containing menthol, phenol, or camphor produce a cool sensation and help reduce itching and burning sensations. Antihistamines such as diphenhydramine, pyrilamine, and tripelennamine relieve itching (see the section on insect stings and bites for more information about topical antihistamines). Topical hydrocortisone is often effective when the above anti-itching agents are not. Do not use topical hydrocortisone on children under age 2. (See the section on topical antibiotics and antiseptics for more information about topical hydrocortisone.)

Astringents

Astringents are effective for drying poison ivy rashes that are blistered or oozing. Effective astringents include aluminum acetate, tannic acid, and zinc oxide. "Shake lotions" such as zinc oxide or calamine (which contains zinc oxide) are widely used as astringents and to reduce itching.

Aluminum acetate solution (Burow's solution) should be applied as a wet dressing 3 to 4 times daily for no longer than 7 days. Packets and tablets of aluminum acetate for mixing the solution at home are available under the brand name Domeboro.

SPECIAL CONSIDERATIONS

Children: Consult a doctor about treating poison ivy in children under age 2.

Poison Ivy Product Cautions

Possible side effects: Some people are sensitive to benzocaine. If your poison ivy rash becomes redder or more itchy after applying a product containing benzocaine, stop using it.

Call Your Doctor:

• If the poison ivy rash covers more than 15 percent of the body.
• If the rash affects the eyes, nose, mouth, respiratory tract, or genital area.
• If the rash is very severe.
• If the rash does not get better or gets worse after 14 days.

POISON IVY PRODUCTS AND COMMON BRANDS

ASTRINGENTS

Brand Name	Application Form	Astringent
Calamine (generic)	lotion	calamine, zinc oxide
Calamox	ointment	calamine
Ivy Dry Liquid	liquid	tannic acid
Obtundia Calamine Cream	cream	calamine, zinc oxide

ANTI-ITCHING AGENTS

Brand Name	Application Form	Anti-Itching Agent
Dermapax	lotion	pyrilamine
Di-Delamine	gel, spray	diphenhydramine
Ivy-Chex	pump spray	methyl salicylate
Pyribenzamine	cream, ointment	tripelennamine
Rhuli Gel	gel	menthol, camphor
Surfadil	lotion	diphenhydramine
Topic	gel	menthol, camphor

ANESTHETICS

Brand Name	Application Form	Anesthetic
Nupercainal	cream, ointment	dibucaine
Pontocaine	cream, ointment	tetracaine
Tronothane Hydrochloride	cream	pramoxine

ANTI-ITCHING AGENT WITH ASTRINGENT

Brand Name	Application Form
Caladryl	cream, lotion
Ziradryl	lotion

ANESTHETIC, ANTI-ITCHING AGENT, AND ASTRINGENT

Brand Name	Application Form
Calamatum	ointment, lotion, spray
Dalicote	lotion
Ivarest	cream, lotion
Ivy Dry	cream
Ivy Super Dry	liquid
Poison Ivy Spray	spray
Rhuli	cream, spray

SLEEP AIDS

When Do You Need a Sleep Aid?

Sleep aids are most often used to relieve occasional insomnia. About one-third of all people sometimes have trouble sleeping. Common causes of simple insomnia include stress and anxiety, pain or discomfort, changes in normal routine or work shift, jet lag, and age. Some prescription and nonprescription drugs contain caffeine or other stimulants, which can prevent sleep. Some prescription drugs, including some sleeping pills, can cause changes in sleep patterns, leading to sleeplessness or bad dreams.

All nonprescription sleep aids contain antihistamines, which have a sedative effect. Some nonprescription sleep aids also contain analgesics to help relieve pain or discomfort.

USING SLEEP AIDS

If you have only occasional trouble sleeping, you probably do not need a sleep aid at all. However, if you are concerned about missing a night's sleep, taking a sleep aid may be a good idea. By definition, sleep aids cause drowsiness. Do not drive, operate hazardous equipment, or do anything requiring mental alertness if you take a sleep aid. Alcohol and other central nervous system depressants may increase the sedative effects of sleep aids and should not be taken with them. Your pharmacist can help you select the brand that is best for you.

TYPES OF SLEEP AIDS

Diphenhydramine

The active ingredient in many sleep aids is diphenhydramine, an antihistamine with a strong sedative effect. The usual dosage for diphenhydramine is 50 mg; it is usually effective within 1 hour. Diphenhydramine is the only nonprescription sleep aid that has been found safe and effective.

Doxylamine

The active ingredient in some sleep aids is doxylamine, an antihistamine with a strong sedative effect. The usual dosage for doxylamine is 25 mg; it is usually effective within 2 hours.

Doxylamine has not been proven to be completely safe and effective, but current regulations allow it to be marketed as a sleep aid and it is unlikely to cause problems. Your pharmacist can answer your questions about this medication.

Combination Sleep Aids

Some sleep aids contain an analgesic, usually acetaminophen, combined with diphenhydramine. These medications help you sleep by relieving pain or discomfort that may be keeping you awake and by the sedative effect of the diphenhydramine.

Other Sleep Aids

The value of sleep aids containing pyrilamine maleate has not been shown and they are not discussed in this book. Your pharmacist can answer your questions about these medications.

The value of the amino acid L-tryptophan as a sleep aid or food supplement has not been shown. In addition, L-tryptophan has been related to a rare and serious blood disorder. Avoid all use of L-tryptophan.

SPECIAL CONSIDERATIONS

Children: Do not give sleep aids to children.

Pregnant and nursing women: Do not use sleep aids if you are pregnant. Sleep aids pass into milk. Avoid them if you are nursing.

Elderly persons: Sensitivity to caffeine increases with age. Instead of a sleep aid, try eliminating caffeine from your diet. Some elderly people have a paradoxical reaction to sleep aids and become more wakeful instead of sleepy. Side effects of sleep aids are more likely to occur in the elderly.

Sleep Aid Abuse

Sleep aids are not habit-forming.

Sleep Aid Overdose

Symptoms of sleep aid overdose include convulsions, hallucinations, red face, and coma. Get medical help immediately.

Cautions for Sleep Aids

Possible side effects: Side effects of sleep aids include dizziness, ringing in the ears, dry mouth and throat, and nausea.

Possible drug interactions: Do not take sleep aids if you also take any sort of central nervous system depressant such a barbiturates or prescription sleeping pills. Do not combine sleep aids and alcohol.

Other medical problems: Avoid sleep aids if you have sleep apnea, asthma, or epilepsy.

Call Your Doctor:

• If you are severely anxious or depressed.

• If you think a prescription medication is causing your sleeplessness.

• If your sleeplessness continues for more than a week.

SLEEP AIDS AND COMMON BRANDS

DIPHENHYDRAMINE

Brand Name	Dose Form
Compoz	tablet
Dormarex 2	tablet
Nervine Night-Time Sleep-Aid	caplet
Nytol	tablet
Sleep-Eze 3	tablet
Sleepinal	tablet
Sominex 2	tablet
Twilite	caplet

DOXYLAMINE

Brand Name	Dose Form
Doxysom	tablet
Unisom Nighttime Sleep Aid	tablet

COMBINATION SLEEP AIDS

Diphenhydramine and Acetaminophen

Brand Name	Dose Form
Excedrin PM	tablet
Sominex Pain Relief Formula	tablet
Tega S-A	tablet

STIMULANTS

When Do You Need a Stimulant?

Nonprescription stimulants are commonly used to help people stay awake and alert during fatiguing situations such as driving long distances at night. Caffeine is the only nonprescription stimulant that has been found to be safe and effective.

USING STIMULANTS

Caffeine is found in chocolate and coffee, tea, and cola drinks. Caffeine is also available in convenient tablet form.

The caffeine content of beverages varies considerably. Five ounces of brewed coffee contains anywhere from 40 to 180 mg of caffeine, depending on the type of coffee and the brewing method. Five ounces of instant coffee contains 30 to 120 mg of caffeine, again depending on the type of coffee. Five ounces of brewed tea contains anywhere from 20 to 110 mg of caffeine, depending on the type of tea and the brewing method. Generally speaking, the stronger or darker the coffee or tea, the more caffeine it contains. Twelve ounces of a cola drink contain anywhere from 36 to 46 mg of caffeine. One ounce of milk chocolate contains 6 mg of caffeine; 1 ounce of dark, semisweet chocolate contains 20 mg of caffeine.

Caffeine tablets generally contain anywhere from 100 to 200 mg of caffeine; some timed-release tablets contain 250 mg. Some pain relievers contain caffeine in addition to the active ingredient. (For more information about these products, see the section on pain relievers.)

In addition to caffeine, some stimulants also contain acetaminophen, sucrose, or dextrose. If you should restrict your intake of any of these ingredients, consult your pharmacist about which product is best for you.

TYPES OF STIMULANTS

Caffeine

Most people drink 2 to 3 cups of coffee every day, in addition to consuming caffeine from other sources. The average adult consumes 210 mg of caffeine daily.

Caffeine can improve alertness and concentration and decrease fatigue. The stimulant effect of caffeine can increase the time it takes to fall asleep and can reduce the quality of sleep. The stimulant effect of caffeine does not counteract the effects of alcohol.

Much controversy surrounds the long-term effects of caffeine. To date, careful studies have failed to find links between caffeine and heart disease, caffeine and cholesterol levels, caffeine and pancreatic, bladder, and breast cancer, and caffeine and benign breast disease. Caffeine may have a slightly adverse effect on individuals with heart arrhythmias, although the evidence is inconclusive.

Dependence on caffeine can develop. Some people routinely consume 600 mg of caffeine on a daily basis. The primary symptom of caffeine withdrawal is a headache; withdrawal symptoms usually disappear within 1 week or less.

SPECIAL CONSIDERATIONS

Children: Do not give stimulants to children.

Pregnant and nursing women: Avoid caffeine during pregnancy and nursing.

Elderly persons: The effects of caffeine may be felt more strongly.

Stimulant Overdose

Symptoms of a caffeine overdose include insomnia, extreme irritability, rapid heartbeat, confusion, fever, convulsions, and coma. Get help immediately.

Cautions for Stimulants

Possible side effects: Consumption of more than 1 gram of caffeine in a day can cause dizziness, restlessness, insomnia, breathlessness, headache, irregular heartbeat, palpitations, and diarrhea. These symptoms are sometimes confused with those of anxiety. In an effort to relieve the headache of caffeine overconsumption, some people take pain relievers. Because these drugs can contain caffeine, they may accidentally make their condition worse instead of better.

Increased urination is an occasional side effect of caffeine.

Possible drug interactions: The effect of caffeine may be felt more by women who take oral contraceptives. Caffeine will decrease the effect of sedatives, tranquilizers, and sleep aids. Do not consume caffeine if you take an MAO inhibitor or an antidepressant medication.

Other medical problems: Avoid caffeine if you have a peptic ulcer, irregular heartbeat, high blood pressure, or hypoglycemia (low blood sugar).

STIMULANTS AND BRAND NAMES

CAFFEINE TABLETS

Brand Name	Caffeine Content
Caffedrine Capsules	200 mg (timed release)
Citrated Caffeine	500 mg
Dexitac Capsules	250 mg (timed release)
NoDoz Tablets	100 mg
Quick-Pep Tablets	150 mg
Summit	100 mg
Tirend Tablets	100 mg
Vivarin Tablets	200 mg
Wakoz	200 mg

TOPICAL ANTIBIOTICS AND ANTISEPTICS

When Do You Need a Topical Antibiotic or Antiseptic?
Topical antibiotics and antiseptics are used to help protect minor cuts, scrapes, and the like from infection. Some topical antibiotics also contain anesthetics to help temporarily relieve discomfort. Topical antibiotics should be used in addition to, not instead of, basic first aid and hygiene.

If the wound is large, deep, jagged or irregular, covers an extensive area, is a deep puncture, or is on the face, get medical help. If the wound spurts blood or does not stop bleeding after several minutes of pressure, it is a medical emergency. Get medical help at once.

Topical antibiotics and antiseptics are meant for external use on the skin only. Do not use these products internally. Do not use them on the eyes, genitals, or anal area, or in the nose, ears, or mouth.

Topical antibiotics and antiseptics can be used to treat minor burns and sunburn, but products specifically designed to provide protection and pain relief for burns and sunburn may be a better choice. (See the section on burns and sunburn for more information.) Although topical antibiotics and antiseptics can be used to treat athlete's foot and other fungal infections, these problems are better treated by antifungal preparations. (See the section athlete's foot and other fungal infections for more information. See the section on poison ivy for more information on treating dermatitis from irritating plants.)

USING TOPICAL ANTIBIOTICS AND ANTISEPTICS

Topical antibiotics or antiseptics should be applied only after a minor skin wound has been properly treated with basic first-aid measures. Minor bleeding from a cut or scrape usually stops by itself after a few minutes. If it does not, place a clean gauze pad over the wound and apply steady pressure for 5 minutes. If bleeding continues after this, get medical help.

Bleeding usually carries away any dirt or debris that may have gotten into a cut or scrape. (A scrape with dirt or grit embedded in it should be cleaned and treated by a physician.) After the bleeding stops, use a clean cotton ball or gauze pad moistened with warm water to clean the area around the wound. Wipe away from the wound. Dry the area. At this point a topical antibiotic or antiseptic may be applied sparingly according to the package directions. Most small cuts and scrapes heal better if they are not bandaged. However, cover the wound with an adhesive bandage strip or gauze if you wish. Minor skin cuts and scrapes generally heal without leaving a scar in about a week.

Topical antibiotics and antiseptics come as ointments, creams, liquids, gels, sprays, and powders. Your choice of topical antibiotic or antiseptic will depend on the active ingredients you prefer and the form you prefer to apply them in. Your pharmacist can help you select the brand that is most appropriate for you.

TYPES OF TOPICAL ANTIBIOTICS AND ANTISEPTICS

Topical Antibiotics

Antibiotics kill bacteria and help prevent infection. The most commonly used antibiotics in nonprescription topical antibiotic products are bacitracin, neomycin, and polymyxin sulfate. Tetracycline is found in a few topical antibiotics.

Bacitracin is available in a number of different dosage forms. It should be applied 1 to 3 times daily. It is safe for topical use on infants and children. Some people develop allergic reactions to bacitracin. Symptoms of hypersensitivity generally include itching, redness, and minor swelling around the wound area. Discontinue the product if a reaction develops.

Neomycin is available as a cream or ointment. It should be applied 1 to 3 times daily. About 8 percent of people who use neomycin develop an allergic reaction to it. Symptoms of hypersensitivity generally include itching, redness, and minor swelling around the wound area. Discontinue the product if a reaction develops.

Polymyxin B sulfate is available in a number of different dose forms. It should be applied 1 to 2 times daily. Allergic reactions of polymyxin are very rare.

Tetracycline, oxytetracycline, and chlortetracycline are all related broad-spectrum antibiotics. Topical antibiotics containing tetracycline should be applied 1 to 3 times daily. Some people are allergic to tetracycline. Symptoms of hypersensitivity include redness, itching, swelling, and hives around the wound area. Discontinue the product if a reaction develops.

Topical Antiseptics

Antiseptics do not kill bacteria. Instead, they slow or inhibit the growth of bacteria that can cause infection. The most commonly used antiseptics in nonprescription topical antibiotic products are iodine, iodophors, mercuric compounds, phenolic compounds, and quaternary ammonium compounds.

Iodine is a well-known antiseptic that has been in use for decades. Iodine can stain skin and fabrics, and it can be irritating to the skin. For this reason, tincture of iodine (2 percent iodine, approximately 50 percent alcohol) is preferred for minor skin injuries. Do not use strong iodine solution (Lugol's solution) on skin wounds. To avoid irritation, don't bandage the wound after applying iodine.

Iodophors such as povidone-iodine are less irritating and less likely to stain than tincture of iodine. The antiseptic effect is more long-lasting.

Mercuric compounds include the well-known mercurochrome. In general, mercuric compounds are not very effective as antiseptics. However, one mercuric compound, thimerosal, is fairly effective and is found in some topical products.

Phenolic compounds include phenol, cresol, resorcinol, hexylresorcinol, and others. In general, phenolic compounds are not very effective as antiseptics. These compounds can be irritating to tissues and should be used in diluted form.

Quaternary ammonium compounds such as benzalkonium chloride are fairly effective as antiseptics and cleansing agents.

Other commonly used antiseptics include ethanol, isopropyl alcohol, and hydrogen peroxide. Ethanol is an effective antiseptic but should be avoided because it is highly irritating to the skin. Isopropyl alcohol is an effective antiseptic and drying agent but it can irritate the skin. Hydrogen peroxide has a cleansing effect on wounds, but does little more. Use hydrogen peroxide when first cleaning a wound but avoid it thereafter. Don't bandage a wound that has been treated with hydrogen peroxide.

Topical Hydrocortisone

Topical hydrocortisone with a 0.50 percent concentration has been available in nonprescription products since 1980. In 1991, topical hydrocortisone at 1 percent concentration was approved for nonprescription sale. Today both 0.50 percent and 1 percent formulations are sold. The brand names are generally the same. The 1 percent formulations are clearly marked as such; in addition, words such as "extra-strength" are often on the packaging.

Hydrocortisone is an effective anti-inflammatory medication for the temporary relief of minor skin irritation, itching, and rashes due to eczema, dermatitis, insect bites, poison ivy, poison oak, and poison sumac. Apply hydrocortisone sparingly to the affected area 3 to 4 times daily. Hydrocortisone products are odorless and do not sting on application. Do not use these products on children under age 2.

SPECIAL CONSIDERATIONS

Children: Topical antibiotics containing bacitracin are generally safe for use on children and infants. Do not treat diaper rash with topical antibiotics. Do not use hydrocortisone on children under age 2.

Cautions for Topical Antibiotics

Possible side effects: Some people are allergic to bacitracin, neomycin, or tetracycline. Symptoms of a reaction include redness, swelling, itching, and hives. Discontinue use of the product if a reaction occurs.

Other medical problems: Skin infections that recur or don't heal rapidly may be a sign of diabetes or other serious problem.

Call Your Doctor:

• If the wound is large, deep, jagged or irregular.
• If the wound covers an extensive area.
• If the wound is a deep puncture.
• If the wound is on the face.
• If the wound spurts blood or keeps bleeding after several minutes of pressure.
• If the wound becomes inflamed or very painful.

- If the wound develops pus or a watery fluid.
- If the wound does not get better or gets worse after 7 days of treatment.

TOPICAL ANTIBIOTICS AND ANTISEPTICS

ANTIBIOTICS WITH BACITRACIN
Brand Name
Baciguent Ointment
Bacitracin (generic)

ANTIBIOTICS WITH TETRACYCLINE
Brand Name
Achromycin Ointment
Aureomycin Ointment

ANTIBIOTICS WITH NEOMYCIN AND POLYMYXIN
Brand Name
Neosporin Cream

ANTIBIOTICS WITH BACITRACIN, NEOMYCIN, AND POLYMYXIN
Brand Name
Bactine First Aid Antibiotic
Lanabiotic Ointment
Medi-Quik
Mycitracin
N.B.P.
Neomixin
Neosporin Ointment
Neosporin Ointment Maximum Strength
Neo-Thrycex
Septa
Trimycin
Triple Antibiotic (generic)
Triple Antibiotic DP
Triple Antibiotic Ointment

ANTIBIOTICS WITH NEOMYCIN
Brand Name
Myciguent Cream
Myciguent Ointment
Neomycin (generic)

ANTIBIOTICS WITH BACITRACIN AND POLYMYXIN
Brand Name
Polysporin Aerosol
Polysporin Ointment
Polysporin Powder

ANTIBIOTICS WITH TETRACYCLINE AND POLYMYXIN
Brand Name
Terramycin Ointment

ANTISEPTICS WITH IODINE
Brand Name
ACU-dyne
Biodine Topical 1%
Efodine
Iodex Regular
Iodine Swabs (generic)
Iodine Topical Solution (generic)
Iodine Tincture (generic)

ANTISEPTICS WITH POVIDONE-IODINE
Brand Name
Betadine Solution
Betadine Swab Sticks
Betadine Gauze Pads
Iodex-P
Isodine Antiseptic Solution
Paladine Solution
Polydine
Povadyne
Poviderm Ointment
Poviderm Solution
Povidone-Iodine (generic

ANTISEPTICS WITH PHENOL OR CRESOL
Brand Name
Campho-Phenique
Obtundia
Obtundia First Aid Spray

ANTISEPTICS WITH
BENZALKONIUM CHLORIDE
Brand Name
Bactine
Benza
Benzalkonium Chloride (generic)
Germicin
Mercurochrome II
Oxyzal Wet Dressing
Zephiran Chloride Solution
Zephiran Chloride Spray
Zephiran Towelettes

ANTISEPTICS WITH RESORCINOL
Brand Name
Castaderm
Castel Minus
Castel Plus
Neo-Castaderm
Oil-O-Sol
S.T. 37

ANTISEPTICS WITH THIMEROSAL
Brand Name
Mersol
Merthiolate Solution
Merthiolate Tincture
Thimerosal (generic)

HYDROCORTISONE PRODUCTS

Brand Name	*Application Form*
Bactine	cream
CaldeCORT	cream, spray
Cortaid	cream, ointment, lotion, spray
Cortizone	cream, ointment
Delacort	lotion
Dermacort	lotion
DermiCort	cream
Dermolate	cream
Dermtex HC	cream
FoilleCort	cream
H_2 Cort	cream
Hydrocortisone (generic)	cream, lotion
Hydro-Tex	cream
Hytone	cream
Lanacort	cream
Pharma-Cort	cream
Racet SE	cream
Rhulicort	cream, lotion

WEIGHT CONTROL

When Do You Need a Weight Control Product?
Nonprescription weight control products are used to help overweight people lose weight on a short-term basis by suppressing the appetite. Weight-control products are not a substitute for more rational and effective ways of losing weight. In the long run, the only way to lose weight is to reduce the number of calories in the diet and get more exercise.

USING WEIGHT CONTROL PRODUCTS

Most weight control products contain phenylpropanolamine, a drug chemically related to ephedrine and amphetamine. Some weight control products also contain a bulk producer, usually carboxymethylcellulose or hydroxypropyl methylcellulose. A few weight control products contain benzocaine.

Dietary aid products such as low-calorie liquid meals and candy-like snacks are not considered drugs and are not discussed in this book. Your doctor or pharmacist can provide more information about these products.

Some weight control products also contain cellulose acetate, stearic acid, various vitamins and minerals, ascorbic acid, caffeine, or grapefruit extract. If you should restrict your intake of any of these ingredients, consult your pharmacist about which product is best for you.

Weight control products come as tablets, capsules, and timed-release capsules. Regular tablets or capsules usually contain 25 mg of phenylpropanolamine and are meant to be taken 3 times a day. Timed release formulations generally contain 75 mg of phenylpropanolamine and are meant to be taken only once a day. Your choice of weight control product will depend on the active ingredients you prefer and the form you prefer to take them in. Your pharmacist can help you select the brand that is most appropriate for you.

TYPES OF WEIGHT CONTROL PRODUCTS

Phenylpropanolamine

Phenylpropanolamine is generally safe and effective for short-term weight control. The maximum daily dose should not exceed 75 mg. Phenylpropanolamine can have side effects, particularly if the recommended dosage is exceeded.

Nonprescription weight control products containing phenylpropanolamine, ephedrine, and caffeine and similar products containing phenylpropanolamine and caffeine have been removed from the market.

Bulk Producers

Some weight control products contain bulk producers such as methylcellulose. The bulk producers supposedly provides a "full" feeling that helps reduce overeating. The effectiveness of this approach to controlling obesity has not been proved, but these products are considered safe. Bulk producers may have an unwanted laxative effect.

Benzocaine

Benzocaine is generally safe and effective for short-term weight control. When taken in small doses in the form of a candy or chewing gum just before meals, benzocaine helps suppress the appetite.

Saccharin

Saccharin is an artificial sweetener with no calories. Dieters who substitute saccharin for sugar can easily remove calories from their diet. Saccharin is a possible carcinogen and may no longer be sold as a sweetener. Regulations still allow saccharin to be used in products specifically labeled as diet foods or drinks.

SPECIAL CONSIDERATIONS

Children: Never give weight control products to children.

Pregnant and nursing women: Do not use any product containing saccharin if you are pregnant. Avoid phenylpropanolamine if you are pregnant or nursing.

Elderly persons: Phenylpropanolamine may cause high blood pressure and heart

problems.
Weight Control Product Abuse
Weight control products can be abused by people excessively concerned about their weight, particularly those who have anorexia or bulimia.
Weight Control Product Overdose
Symptoms of an overdose of phenylpropanolamine include anxiety, confusion, delirium, muscle tremors, and rapid pulse. Get medical help immediately.
Cautions for Weight Control Products
Possible side effects: Side effects of phenylpropanolamine include nervousness, restlessness, insomnia, nausea, headache, and high blood pressure. A side effect of bulk producers may be diarrhea.
Possible drug interactions: Phenylpropanolamine is also found in some nonprescription asthma, cold, cough, and allergy medications. If you take another medication containing phenylpropanolamine, do not also take a weight control product containing the drug. Do not take phenylpropanolamine if you also take an antidepressant, an MAO inhibitor, or medication for high blood pressure or a heart condition. Avoid caffeine and alcoholic beverages.
Other medical problems: Avoid phenylpropanolamine if you have high blood pressure, heart disease, diabetes, thyroid problems, or prostate problems.
Call Your Doctor:
• If you have difficulty urinating.

WEIGHT CONTROL PRODUCTS AND COMMON BRANDS

PHENYLPROPANOLAMINE

Brand Name	Dose Level	Other Ingredients
Appedrine Tablets	25 mg	vitamins and minerals
Control	75 mg	
Dex-A-Diet Extended Release	75 mg	
Dex-A-Diet Maximum Strength	75 mg	
Dex-A-Diet with Vitamin C Capsules	75 mg	ascorbic acid
Dexatrim Capsules	50 mg	
Dexatrim Maximum Strength	75 mg	
Dexatrim Plus Vitamin C Maximum Strength	75 mg	
Dexatrim Pre-Meal	25 mg	ascorbic acid
Dexatrim Caffeine Free Maximum Strength	75 mg	
Grapefruit Plan with Diadex	30 mg	
Grapefruit Plan with Diadex Extra Strength	75 mg	grapefruit extract
Grapefruit Plan with Diadex Extra Strength Vitamin Fortified	75 mg	grapefruit extract
Phenoxine	25 mg	grapefruit extract, ascorbic acid, Vitamin E
Prolamine	38 mg	
Super Odrinex	25 mg	caffeine
Thinz Back-To-Nature	75 mg	
Thinz Before Meals	25 mg	caffeine, other
Thinz Drops	25 mg	ascorbic acid, other
Thinz-Span	75 mg	fructose, other
Unitrol	75 mg	caffeine, other

PHENYLPROPANOLAMINE WITH BULK PRODUCER	
Brand Name	*Dose Level*
Accutrim 16 Hour Steady Control	75 mg
Accutrim Late Day Tablets	75 mg
Accutrim II Maximum Strength Tablets	75 mg

BENZOCAINE	
Brand Name	*Dose Level*
Diet Ayds	6 mg

PHENYLPROPANOLAMINE WITH BULK PRODUCER AND BENZOCAINE		
Brand Name	*Dose Level*	*Benzocaine Dose Level*
Diet-Trim	not specified	not specified
Dieutrim T.D.	75 mg	9 mg

YEAST INFECTIONS

Yeast infection medications treat and cure the vaginal itching, burning, and discharge of vaginal yeast infections (candidiasis or moniliasis).

Vaginal yeast infections are very common. Nearly 13 million American women suffer from vaginal yeast infections yearly; 75 percent of all women will experience a yeast infection at least once in their lives. At least 37 percent of those women who get a yeast infection will get another one. Some women are more susceptible to yeast infections and may have 2 or more infections in a year.

Most yeast infections are caused by an excessive amount of the yeast organism known as *Candida albicans* in the vagina. This yeast organism is naturally present in most women and usually causes no problems. Sometimes, however, the yeast can grow very quickly and cause candidiasis.

A yeast infection can occur at almost any time of life. It is most common, however, during the childbearing years. Yeast infections tend to develop most often in women who are pregnant, diabetic, taking antibiotics, or taking oral contraceptives (birth control pills). Douching can disturb the vaginal balance and lead to yeast infections.

If you are susceptible to yeast infections, it is a good idea to avoid factors that can lead to an infection by allowing yeast to grow. Avoid tight jeans, nylon underwear, pantyhose, damp exercise clothing, and wet swimsuits; these trap moisture and warmth in the genital region and allow yeast to grow rapidly. Cutting down on sweets, milk products, and artificial sweeteners sometimes helps to reduce the incidence of yeast infections. Good personal hygiene also helps.

Consult your doctor about having sexual intercourse when you have a yeast infection. If your partner develops penile itching, redness, or discomfort, he should see a doctor and mention that you are being treated for a yeast infection.

USING YEAST INFECTION MEDICATIONS

If you have never been treated for a yeast infection, see your doctor if you develop the symptoms of candidiasis. If your doctor has already diagnosed you at least once before as having a yeast infection, you will probably recognize the symptoms immediately if they recur. Yeast infection symptoms include: vaginal itching (ranging from mild to intense); a clumpy, white vaginal discharge that may resemble cottage cheese; vaginal soreness, irritation, or burning, particularly during intercourse; and a rash or redness around the vagina. If your symptoms do not resemble these, you may have some other sort of infection. Consult your doctor.

If you are certain that you have a yeast infection again, and if you are certain you are not pregnant, self-treatment with an antifungal medication may be appropriate for you.

Safe and effective antifungal medications for yeast infections have been available without a prescription since 1991. These medications are available as creams or suppositories that are inserted into the vagina once a day using the applicator included with the medication. It is important to follow the manufacturer's instructions precisely and to complete the full 7-day course of treatment. Often the symptoms of a yeast infection disappear very quickly when treatment begins. If treatment is stopped too early, however, the symptoms will return.

Yeast infection medications can be used during menstruation. Do not use tampons, however, since they can absorb the medication. Use sanitary pads or napkins instead.

TYPES OF YEAST INFECTION MEDICATIONS

Miconazole Nitrate

Miconazole nitrate is an antifungal that is the active ingredient in Monistat 7. This medication has been available on a nonprescription basis since 1991. Monistat 7 relieves symptoms rapidly and can cure most yeast infections. It is available in cream and vaginal suppository form.

Clotrimazole

Clotrimazole is an antifungal that is the active ingredient in Gyne-Lotrimin. This medication has been available on a nonprescription basis since 1991. Gyne-Lotrimin relieves symptoms rapidly and can cure most yeast infections. It is available in cream and vaginal suppository form.

Hydrocortisone

Several products designed to relieve "feminine itching" contain hydrocortisone. These products only relieve symptoms; they do not treat the underlying problem. Although these products are safe and effective, they can mask the symptoms of yeast infections or other types of vaginal infections. See your doctor if you have vaginal itching and do not know why.

Products containing hydrocortisone include Cortef Feminine Itch Cream, Gynecort Creme, Massengill Medicated Towelettes, and Vagisil. Another, Vaginex Cream, contains tripelennamine, an antihistamine that helps relieve itching.

SPECIAL CONSiDERATIONS
Pregnant and nursing women: Yeast infections are very common during pregnancy. Discuss the problem with your doctor before using a nonprescription product.
Diabetics: Careful control of diabetes may help prevent yeast infections. Discuss the problem with your doctor before using a nonprescription product.
Call Your Doctor:
• If you have never had a yeast infection before.
• If your yeast infection symptoms do not improve after 3 days of using a nonprescription antifungal.
• If your yeast infection is not completely relieved after 7 days of using a nonprescription antifungal.
• If you are or think you might be pregnant.
• If you have diabetes.

INTRODUCTION

WHAT ARE VITAMINS AND MINERALS?

Vitamins are organic substances needed in very small amounts to sustain life. Not enough of all the vitamins needed to sustain a healthy human are produced within the body. Instead, we get most of the vitamins we need from the food we eat. Minerals are chemical substances, such as calcium and potassium, found in the human body. They are essential for such important body functions as building bones and conducting nerve impulses. As with vitamins, we get most of the minerals we need from the food we eat.

There are 11 vitamins essential for the human body. Vitamins fall into two categories: fat-soluble and water-soluble. The fat-soluble vitamins are Vitamins A, D, E, and K. The water-soluble vitamins are Vitamins C and the various B vitamins, including thiamin, riboflavin, niacin, Vitamin B_6, folate, and Vitamin B_{12}.

Fat-soluble vitamins are absorbed into the body along with fats. These vitamins are found in the fat or oil of foods. Fat-soluble vitamins are generally stored by the body in the tissues. Water-soluble vitamins are found in the watery parts of foods. They are more likely to be destroyed or lost when food is cooked. These vitamins are not stored by the body; if you take in more than your body needs, the excess is excreted.

Vitamins are generally found in two forms: preformed compounds, which contain the vitamin itself, and "building block" or protovitamin compounds, which are converted into the vitamin by the body. For example, Vitamin A is found as the preformed compounds retinal and retinol in animal foods such as eggs. The protovitamin compound beta carotene, which is found in dark green vegetables such as kale, is converted into Vitamin A by the body when it is ingested.

There are numerous minerals needed by the human body. Of these, 7 are considered major minerals (that is, a typical human body contains more than 1 teaspoon of the mineral). The rest are considered "trace" minerals because the typical human body contains less than 1 teaspoon of each. However, trace minerals are just as important for normal body functions are major minerals are.

RECOMMENDED DIETARY ALLOWANCES (RDAS)

Recommended Dietary Allowances (RDAs) of vitamins and minerals have been set by the independent National Research Council since 1941. Recommended Dietary Allowances are the levels of intake of essential nutrients that, on the basis of scientific knowledge, are judged by the Food and Nutrition Board of the National Research Council to be adequate to meet the known nutrient needs of practically all healthy persons.

RDAs for individuals depend on their age, sex, height, and weight. RDAs for adult women vary if the woman is pregnant or nursing. The RDAs take into account nutrient losses due to food processing and cooking. Other factors, such as occasional minor illness and occasional poor nutrition, are taken into account by the RDAs. If anything, the RDAs err on the side of generosity. For example, the amount of calcium in the RDA is the amount recommended for young women, who have the highest need for this mineral. Most young men need less than the RDA for calcium.

When deciding if you have met your RDA for vitamins and minerals, remember to count both the amounts you ingest through food and the amounts you ingest through supplements.

SUPPLEMENTS AND NUTRITION

Most nutrition experts agree that most people can obtain all the vitamins and minerals they need by eating a well-balanced, normal diet—that is, a diet that contains a variety of foods from different food groups. If you are in good health and eat a balanced diet on a fairly regular basis, you probably don't need foods "fortified" with vitamins and minerals or vitamin and mineral supplements. However, not everyone is in good health all the time, and not everyone can eat properly all the time. If you are concerned about meeting your RDAs, you may wish to take supplemental vitamins and minerals. Remember, however, that supplements are not a substitute for a good diet. If you are pregnant or nursing, or if you have a serious illness, injury, or chronic disease, your doctor may prescribe supplemental vitamins. Doctors may recommend nonprescription supplemental vitamins for infants and children. If you wish to take vitamins on a nonprescription basis, or if you wish to give vitamins to infants and children, discuss the subject with your doctor first.

Vitamins and minerals have no calories. The amount of vitamins and minerals in foods can vary, depending on the type of food and how it is stored and prepared. In general, fresh foods and foods that have not been overcooked have the highest vitamin and mineral contents.

READING THE LABELS

The federal Food and Drug Administration treats vitamins and minerals as food supplements, not drugs. Manufacturers are not allowed to make health claims for their products. The RDAs set by the National Research Council are the basis for the guidelines used in the nutritional labeling of food, which is required by the Food and Drug Administration. All this gives rise to some confusion, because the labeling on food packages and food supplements (including vitamin and mineral supplements) gives the nutrient content in terms of U.S. Recommended Daily Allowances (USRDAs), which are set by the FDA. USRDAs and RDAs are virtually identical.

USRDAs are usually expressed on the label as a percentage of the total. The label on a container of vitamin supplements lists the amount of each ingredient in both units (30 mg, for example) and as a percentage of the U.S. Recommended Daily Allowance (100, for example).

Proposals under consideration by the FDA would change the term USRDA to a new term for dietary standards, the Reference Daily Intake, or RDI. The RDI requirements would be based on the levels needed by average individuals and thus would tend to be lower than the USRDAs, which are based on the levels needed by people with the highest, not the average, requirement. The RDI proposals are controversial and still under discussion.

The measurement of vitamins and minerals can be a little confusing. Only very small amounts of vitamins and minerals are needed by the body. The units used to express the amounts needed can vary from substance to substance. In general, the amounts of vitamins and minerals are expressed as milligrams (mg), micrograms (mcg), or International Units (IU). A milligram (mg) is a metric weight unit that is 1/1,1000th of a gram (a gram is equivalent to 1/28th of an ounce). A microgram (mcg) is even smaller; it is equivalent to 1/1,000 of a milligram, or one millionth of a gram. An International Unit is an arbitrary unit of measurement used for vitamins A, D, and E. It does not measure the weight of the vitamin; instead, it indicates the potency (biological activity) of the vitamin. The IU measurement can be converted to mg or mcg equivalents (see the sections on vitamins A, D, and E for more information).

The labels of vitamin and mineral supplements contain other important information. All the ingredients in supplements are listed; if no minerals are listed on the label, the product contains only vitamins. Just as with nonprescription drugs, the label gives the name and location of the manufacturer or packer, the expiration date and lot or batch number, a description of tamper-resistant features, recommended dosages, and more. (See the introduction to this book for more information about labels and using and storing nonprescription drugs. Much of this information applies to vitamin and mineral supplements as well.)

CHOOSING SUPPLEMENTS

A confusing variety of vitamin and mineral supplements is available today. In general, however, supplements fall into two categories: single ingredient and multiple ingredient.

Single-ingredient supplements are just that: supplements that contain only one particular vitamin or mineral. Multi-ingredient supplements usually contain a number of vitamins and minerals. Also known as multivitamins, multi-ingredient supplements often contain many vitamins and minerals (as many as 20 or more) in doses that are often at least as large as the RDA. Some multivitamin formulas claim to be "high-potency" or "stress" formulas. These formulas contain more of the vitamins you supposedly need if you are under stress, don't have the time to eat properly, and so on. There is little evidence that these formulations have any more positive effect than other formulations.

Many single-ingredient and multi-ingredient vitamin supplements contain more of the vitamins and minerals than the RDA. Is more better? Not necessarily. In the case of water-soluble vitamins, the excess is simply excreted. In the case of fat-soluble vitamins, some of the excess is excreted and some is stored in the tissues. Too much of some fat-soluble vitamins (Vitamin A, for example) can be dangerous. Excess minerals are generally excreted. Very large doses of some minerals can be dangerous.

Some vitamins are advertised as being "organic." This is said to mean that the vitamins come from "natural" sources—Vitamin C from rose hips, for example. Organic vitamins tend to be somewhat more expensive than "regular" vitamins. Vitamins, however, are basically complex chemical molecules; a Vitamin C molecule is exactly the same whether it is derived from rose hips or made in a laboratory. In addition, there is little that is natural about the process of making organic vitamins. Powerful chemical solvents are used to separate the vitamins from the organic source. Consumers should be very wary of the "organic" claim.

Brand-name vitamin supplements are heavily advertised. These brands are good products, but they are generally more expensive than equally good generic and lesser-known brands. Ask your pharmacist to help you compare brands and select the one that is the best for you and your budget.

TAKING SUPPLEMENTS

The manufacturers of many vitamin supplements (especially multivitamins) suggest taking one tablet daily. There is probably no harm in doing so, although you will probably simply excrete many of the ingredients. Some manufacturers produce "timed-release" or "long-lasting" supplements. The idea behind these is that the vitamins are released gradually as the tablet passes through your digestive system; this is said to help maintain a constant level of needed vitamins. There is little evidence to support the claims for timed-release tablets. In fact, you may actually absorb less of the vitamins by taking these tablets. Some vitamins and minerals are absorbed into the body only at specific points in the digestive system. If a particular vitamin is not released at the particular absorption point, it will simply pass through and out of your body.

Vitamin and mineral supplements are available as pills, tablets, chewable tablets, capsules, gelcaps, and liquids. Many chewable tablets, especially those for children, contain sucrose, fructose, glucose, or saccharin as a sweetener. Many multi-ingredient formulas are in the form of large tablets. If you have difficulty swallowing these tablets, you can break them in half or crush them and take them with food. Supplements vary considerably in their formulation. Some contain a single vitamin or mineral; others contain several; still others contain many. Your pharmacist can help you choose the dose form and formulation that are most appropriate for you.

VITAMIN A

What Vitamin A Does for You

Vitamin A is a fat-soluble vitamin needed for normal growth and health and for healthy eyes and skin. Eye problems such as night blindness are the most likely symptoms of Vitamin A deficiency. Vitamin A was the first vitamin to be discovered, in 1913.

Vitamin A occurs naturally in several different forms, or compounds. The most common compounds of Vitamin A are retinol, retinal, and carotenoids.

Retinol and retinal are compounds found naturally in certain foods; they contain preformed Vitamin A. Carotenoids are compounds found naturally in certain foods; they contain beta carotene, a protovitamin that is converted to Vitamin A in the body.

RDAS FOR VITAMIN A

The measurement units for Vitamin A are a little confusing. The terms Retinol Equivalent (RE) and micrograms (mcg) of retinol are used interchangeably. One RE is equal to 1 mcg of retinol. The term International Unit (IU) is also used for Vitamin A. One mcg of Vitamin A is the equivalent of 3.33 IU. However, because the average person gets somewhat more than half the required Vitamin A as the protovitamin beta carotene, for RDA purposes it is assumed that 1 RE is equivalent to 5 IU.

RDAS FOR VITAMIN A		
Age in years	*Daily RE/mcg*	*Daily IU*
birth to 1	375	1875
1 to 3	400	2000
4 to 6	500	2500
7 to 10	700	3500
11+ males	1000	5000
11+ females	800	4000
pregnant	800	4000
nursing, 1st 6 months	1300	6500
nursing, 2nd 6 months	1200	6000

DIETARY SOURCES OF VITAMIN A

Preformed Vitamin A is found in animal foods such as liver, kidneys, eggs, cream, whole milk, butter, and whole-milk cheese. Beta carotene is found in orange, dark yellow, and dark green fruits and vegetables; the darker or deeper the color, the higher the beta carotene content. Beta carotene is found in collard greens, beet greens, spinach, kale, chard, broccoli, carrots, sweet potatoes, squash, apricots, peaches, cantaloupes, and other fruits and vegetables.

CAUTIONS FOR VITAMIN A

Excess preformed Vitamin A accumulates in the body. If large amounts of preformed Vitamin A (over 50,000 IU daily for adults; over 25,000 IU daily for children) are taken over long periods, toxicity can develop. Symptoms of Vitamin

A toxicity include nausea, vomiting, headaches, bone and joint pain, and cracked lips. In animal studies, birth defects occurred when overdoses of Vitamin A were given. The symptoms of Vitamin A overdose usually go away quickly when excessive intake is stopped. It is almost impossible to overdose on beta carotene because it is not toxic. If extremely large amounts of foods containing beta carotene are consumed, a harmless yellowing of the skin may occur. This symptom usually goes away quickly when excessive intake is stopped.

VITAMIN B COMPLEX
What B Vitamins Do for You
The Vitamin B complex consists of a number of different, but related compounds. All are important for converting food to energy in the body and for maintaining the proper functioning of the nervous system.

VITAMIN B_1 (THIAMIN)
What Vitamin B_1 Does for You
Vitamin B_1, also called thiamin, is a water-soluble vitamin needed for the normal functioning of all body cells, especially the nerves. The most common symptom of thiamin deficiency is beriberi, a disease seen very rarely in the United States. Less severe forms of thiamin deficiency are seen in people with severe illnesses, severe burns, liver disease, alcoholism, and some other conditions. People using artificial kidneys (hemodialysis) can also have thiamin deficiency.

RDAS FOR VITAMIN B_1 (THIAMIN)
The body does not store thiamin; any excess is excreted in the urine. Thiamin is measured in milligrams (mg).

RDAS FOR VITAMIN B_1 (THIAMIN)	
Age in years	*Daily mg*
birth to 6 months	0.3
6 months to 1	0.4
1 to 3	0.7
4 to 6	0.9
7 to 10	1.0
11 to 14 males	1.1
11 to 50 females	1.1
15 to 50 males	1.5
50+ females	1.0
50+ males	1.2
pregnant	1.5
nursing	1.6

DIETARY SOURCES OF VITAMIN B_1 (THIAMIN)
Thiamin is found in many foods. Organ meats, beef, and pork are high in thiamin. Other good sources of thiamin are green peas, dried beans and peas, whole grains, wheat germ, brewer's yeast, peanuts, peanut butter, nuts, collard greens, and oranges. Many grain, cereal, and bakery products are fortified with thiamin.

CAUTIONS FOR VITAMIN B₁ (THIAMIN)

Because thiamin is water-soluble, it does not build up in the body and cause toxicity. If your doctor has prescribed thiamin for you, discuss potential problems with him or her.

VITAMIN B₂ (RIBOFLAVIN)

What Vitamin B₂ (Riboflavin) Does for You

Vitamin B₂, also called riboflavin, is a water-soluble vitamin needed for the normal functions of all body cells. Riboflavin is also important for the normal release of energy from food, for the production of red blood cells, and for the production of some hormones. The most common symptoms of riboflavin deficiency are itchy, burning eyes, sensitivity to light, peeling skin, and sores in the mouth. Riboflavin deficiency is quite rare in the United States. Less severe forms of riboflavin deficiency are seen in people with severe illnesses, severe burns, liver disease, overactive thyroid, and some other conditions. Infants with high blood levels of bilirubin are sometimes given riboflavin.

RDAS FOR VITAMIN B₂ (RIBOFLAVIN)

The body does not store riboflavin; any excess is excreted in the urine, giving it a harmless fluorescent yellow color. Riboflavin is measured in milligrams (mg).

RDAS FOR VITAMIN B₂ (RIBOFLAVIN)	
Age in years	*Daily mg*
birth to 6 months	0.4
6 months to 1	0.5
1 to 3	0.8
4 to 6	1.1
7 to 10	1.2
11 to 14 females	1.4
11 to 14 males	1.7
15+ males	2.0
15 to 18 females	1.5
19+ females	1.6
pregnant	2.2
nursing	2.1

DIETARY SOURCES OF VITAMIN B₂ (RIBOFLAVIN)

Riboflavin in found in many foods. Milk and milk products are high in riboflavin. Other good sources of thiamin are green leafy vegetables such as spinach and collard greens, broccoli, Brussels sprouts, asparagus, avocados, and mushrooms. Canned salmon and beef liver are other sources of riboflavin.

CAUTIONS FOR VITAMIN B₂ (RIBOFLAVIN)

Because riboflavin is water-soluble, it does not build up in the body and cause toxicity. If your doctor has prescribed riboflavin for you, discuss potential problems with him or her.

NIACIN

What Niacin Does for You

Niacin is a water-soluble vitamin that is part of the Vitamin B family. Niacin is needed for the normal functioning of all body cells, especially the release of energy from food and the formation of red blood cells. Humans can synthesize niacin in the body from tryptophan, another substance found in food. The most common symptom of niacin deficiency is pellagra, a disease seen very rarely in the United States. Less severe forms of niacin deficiency are seen in people with cancer, diabetes, severe illnesses, liver disease, overactive thyroid, and some other conditions.

RDAS FOR NIACIN

The body does not store niacin; any excess is excreted in the urine. Niacin is measured in milligrams (mg).

RDAS FOR NIACIN	
Age in years	*Daily mg*
birth to 6 months	5
6 months to 1	6
1 to 3	9
4 to 6	12
7 to 10	13
11 to 14 males	17
15 to 18 males	20
19 to 50 males	19
50+ males	15
11 to 50 females	15
50+ females	13
pregnant	17
nursing	20

DIETARY SOURCES OF NIACIN

Niacin or the protovitamin tryptophan are found in protein-rich foods, including animal foods such as meat, chicken, fish, eggs, low-fat and non-fat milk, and cheese. Vegetable sources of niacin and tryptophan include dried beans and peas, brewer's yeast, orange juice, peanut butter, nuts, and soybeans. Many grain, cereal, and bakery products are fortified with niacin.

CAUTIONS FOR NIACIN

Because niacin is water-soluble, it does not build up in the body and cause toxicity. If your doctor has prescribed niacin for you, discuss potential problems with him or her.

VITAMIN B$_6$

What Vitamin B$_6$ Does for You

Vitamin B$_6$, also called pyridoxine, is a water-soluble vitamin needed for the normal functioning of the carbohydrates, fats, and proteins in the body. Vitamin B$_6$ is essential for converting and synthesizing amino acids, for converting tryptophan to niacin, for proper functioning of the nervous system, and for manufacturing hormones in the body. Symptoms of severe Vitamin B_6 deficiency are sometimes similar to those of pellagra, but this is very rare in the United States. The symptoms of less severe Vitamin B_6 deficiency include nausea, vomiting, depression, dermatitis, anemia, and kidney stones. Vitamin B_6 deficiency are sometimes seen in women who are pregnant or taking oral contraceptives. People who are undergoing radiation treatment, people taking some drugs such as chlorpromazine, and alcoholics may have symptoms of Vitamin B_6 deficiency.

RDAS FOR VITAMIN B_6

Vitamin B_6 is measured in milligrams (mg).

RDAS FOR VITAMIN B_6	
Age in years	Daily mg
birth to 6 months	0.3
6 months to 1	0.6
1 to 3	1.0
4 to 6	1.1
7 to 10	1.4
11 to 14 females	1.4
11 to 14 males	1.7
15 to 18 females	1.5
15+ males	2.0
19+ females	1.6
pregnant	2.2
nursing	2.1

DIETARY SOURCES OF VITAMIN B_6

Vitamin B_6 is found in many foods. Animal foods such as meat, poultry, and fish are high in Vitamin B_6, as are brewer's yeast, dried beans and peas, soybeans, and peanuts. Moderately good dietary sources of Vitamin B_6 include bananas, dried fruits, cabbage, cauliflower, avocados, and potatoes. Many grain, cereal, and bakery products are fortified with Vitamin B_6.

CAUTIONS FOR VITAMIN B_6

Although Vitamin B_6 is water-soluble, it can quickly be toxic when taken in very large doses of greater than 2,000 mg per day. Lower doses of 200 mg per day can be toxic if continued over a long period. If your doctor has prescribed Vitamin B_6 for you, discuss potential problems with him or her.

VITAMIN B_{12}

What Vitamin B_{12} Does for You

Vitamin B_{12} (also called cobalamin) is a water-soluble vitamin needed for the proper metabolization of carbohydrates, protein, and fat in the body. It is also important for the proper functioning of the nervous system. Most importantly, Vitamin B_{12} is important for healthy blood. Humans must obtain all their Vitamin B_{12} from the foods they eat. Pernicious anemia, which develops in some adults whose intestines stop absorbing Vitamin B_{12}, can be cured by taking prescription-strength Vitamin B_{12}. Symptoms of less severe Vitamin B_{12} deficiency include anemia and nerve damage.

RDAS FOR VITAMIN B_{12}

Vitamin B_{12} is measured in micrograms (mcg). Humans need very little Vitamin B_{12}.

RDAS FOR VITAMIN B_{12}	
Age in years	Daily mcg
birth to 6 months	0.3
6 months to 1	0.5
1 to 3	0.7
4 to 6	1.0
7 to 10	1.4
11+	2.0
pregnant	2.2
nursing	2.1

DIETARY SOURCES OF VITAMIN B_{12}

Vitamin B_{12} is found only in animal foods and foods that have been fermented. Good sources of Vitamin B_{12} include meat, poultry, organ meats, fish, shellfish, eggs, milk and cheese.

CAUTIONS FOR VITAMIN B_{12}

Because Vitamin B_{12} is water-soluble, it does not build up in the body and cause toxicity even at many times the RDA. If your doctor has prescribed Vitamin B_{12} for you, discuss potential problems with him or her.

FOLATE (FOLIC ACID)

What Folate (Folic Acid) Does for You

Folate (folic acid) is a water-soluble compound that helps the body control genetic material and regulate cell division. The most common symptom of folate deficiency is impaired cell division. This has the greatest effect on the blood; thus anemia is also a symptom of folate deficiency. People who have serious illnesses, intestinal disease, liver disease, alcoholism, or are using artificial kidneys (hemodialysis) can also have symptoms of folate deficiency.

RDAS FOR FOLATE

The body stores folate only in small amounts in the liver and other tissues; the rest is excreted in the urine. Folate is measured in micrograms (mcg).

RDAS FOR FOLATE (FOLIC ACID)	
Age in years	Daily mcg
birth to 6 months	25
6 months to 1	35
1 to 3	50
4 to 6	75
7 to 10	100
11 to 14 female	200
11 to 14 male	150

15+ female	180
15+ male	200
pregnant	400
nursing, 1st 6 months	280
nursing, 2nd 6 months	260

DIETARY SOURCES OF FOLATE
Folate is found in leafy green vegetables such as spinach and lettuce and in other vegetables such as broccoli, potatoes, avocados, brussels sprouts, beans, and beets. Other vegetable sources include brewer's yeast, orange juice, and bananas. Folate is also found in organ meats, grains, and cereal products.

CAUTIONS FOR FOLATE
Because very little folate is stored in the body, toxicity is unlikely to develop even if you take many times the RDA. If your doctor has prescribed folate for you, discuss potential problems with him or her.

OTHER B VITAMINS
Biotin, also called Vitamin B_7, and pantothenic acid, also called Vitamin B_3, are important to numerous body functions. These vitamins are found in many foods that contain other B vitamins and only very small amounts are needed.

VITAMIN C
What Vitamin C Does for You
Vitamin C (ascorbic acid) is a water-soluble vitamin that is crucial for making and maintaining collagen, the tough substance that forms connective tissue in the body. Humans cannot synthesize Vitamin C; all the Vitamin C the body needs must come from the diet. Severe Vitamin C deficiency causes scurvy, a disease that was once common among sailors on long ocean voyages. Symptoms of scurvy include bleeding gums, loose teeth, swollen joints, and aching muscles. Scurvy is very rare in the United States today.

RDAS FOR VITAMIN C
A minimum of 10 milligrams (mg) of Vitamin C a day are needed to prevent scurvy. People who smoke should ingest at least 100 mg a day because tobacco smoke interferes with the body's ability to absorb Vitamin C. The body does not store Vitamin C; any excess is excreted in the urine. Vitamin C is measured in milligrams (mg).

RDAS FOR VITAMIN C	
Age in years	*Daily mg*
birth to 6 months	30
6 months to 1	35
1 to 3	40
4 to 10	45
11 to 14	50
15+	60
pregnant	70
nursing, 1st 6 months	95
nursing, 2nd 6 months	90

DIETARY SOURCES OF VITAMIN C

Vitamin C is found in citrus fruits such as oranges, tangerines, grapefruits, lemons, and limes. Green vegetables such as broccoli, cabbage, and peppers contain Vitamin C; tomatoes and potatoes are also good sources. There is very little Vitamin C in animal foods such as milk or meat and in grains and nuts.

CAUTIONS FOR VITAMIN C

Many claims have been made for the benefits of very large doses of Vitamin C. There is no scientific evidence that Vitamin C helps treat or cure the common cold, cancer, or any other illness except scurvy. Because Vitamin C is water-soluble, it does not build up in the body and cause toxicity. However, very large doses of Vitamin C (greater than 1 gram daily) over a long period could cause toxicity.

VITAMIN D

What Vitamin D Does for You

Vitamin D is a fat-soluble vitamin needed for proper utilization of calcium by the body, including building bones and regulating the level of calcium in the blood. The most common symptom of Vitamin D deficiency is rickets, a childhood disease that leads to weak and malformed bones.

Vitamin D occurs naturally in three different forms: D_1, D_2, and D_3. Vitamins D_1 and D_2 are found in certain foods. Vitamin D_3 is synthesized in the body by the skin after exposure to sunlight; the other forms of Vitamin D are found in certain foods.

RDAS FOR VITAMIN D

Vitamin D is measured in International Units (IU) or micrograms (mcg). One mcg of Vitamin D is the equivalent of 40 IU. Because most people get enough Vitamin D through exposure to sunlight, it is difficult to establish an RDA for dietary Vitamin D.

RDAS FOR VITAMIN D		
Age in years	*Daily mcg*	*Daily IU*
birth to 6 months	7.5	300
6 months to 10	10	400
11 to 25	10	400
25+	5	200
pregnant	10	400
nursing	10	400

DIETARY SOURCES OF VITAMIN D

Fortified milk containing Vitamin D is the primary dietary source for most Americans. One quart of milk (whole, low-fat, or no-fat) contains 400 IU of Vitamin D. Dairy products such as cheese and yogurt do not usually contain Vitamin D because they are not usually made using fortified milk. By the same token, raw milk and goat milk and products made from them do not contain Vitamin D. Other sources of Vitamin D are liver, eggs, cod liver oil, other fish oils, shrimp, and fish such as canned sardines and fresh mackerel, herring, and salmon. Most plant foods are very low in Vitamin D.

CAUTIONS FOR VITAMIN D

Excess dietary Vitamin D (more than 4 times the RDA) can be toxic (exposure to sunlight does not cause Vitamin D toxicity). Symptoms of Vitamin D toxicity include diarrhea, nausea, headaches, and calcium deposits in soft tissue. The symptoms usually go away quickly when excessive intake is stopped. Calcium deposits, however, may cause irreversible tissue damage.

VITAMIN E

What Vitamin E Does for You

Vitamin E is a fat-soluble vitamin needed as an antioxidant in the body. Free radicals (unattached oxygen molecules) in the body can oxidize, or damage, cells in the body. Vitamin E prevents this from happening. Specifically, Vitamin E protects the cells and tissue from damage, helps regulate and use Vitamin A, and protects the red blood cells from damage. Hemolytic anemia and nerve damage are symptoms of Vitamin E deficiency; however, an actual deficiency of Vitamin E is very rare.

Vitamin E occurs naturally in several different forms. The most active form is known as alpha tocopherol, or sometimes just tocopherol. Synthetic Vitamin E is known as dl-alpha tocopherol; natural Vitamin E is known as d-alpha tocopherol.

RDAS FOR VITAMIN E

Vitamin E is measured in International Units (IU) of alpha-tocopherol or milligrams (mg). One IU of dl-alpha tocopherol (synthetic Vitamin E) is the equivalent of 1 mg; 1.49 IU of d-alpha tocopherol (natural Vitamin E) is the equivalent of 1 mg. In the chart below, the IU is given in terms of dl-alpha tocopherol (synthetic Vitamin E); therefore, the daily RDA is the same in both mg and IU.

RDAS FOR VITAMIN E	
Age in years	*Daily mg/IU*
0 to 6 months	3
6 months to 1	4
1 to 3	6
4 to 10	7
11+ males	10
11+ females	8
pregnant	10
nursing, 1st 6 months	12
nursing, 2nd 6 months	11

DIETARY SOURCES OF VITAMIN E

Vitamin E is found in vegetable oils (particularly sunflower oil and safflower oil), wheat germ, whole grains, and nuts. Green leafy vegetables such as spinach and broccoli are high in Vitamin E. Other dietary sources of Vitamin E are asparagus, avocadoes, peaches, and dried prunes. Most animal foods such as meat and milk are low in Vitamin E.

CAUTIONS FOR VITAMIN E

Little is known about Vitamin E toxicity. Extremely high doses could interfere with the activity of other vitamins. In general, because fat-soluble vitamins accumulate in the body, avoid large doses of Vitamin E.

VITAMIN K
What Vitamin K Does for You
Vitamin K is a fat-soluble vitamin that regulates normal blood clotting by aiding in the production of prothrombin, a protein needed for clotting. The most common symptom of Vitamin K deficiency is clotting problems, but Vitamin K deficiency is very rare. Prolonged antibiotic therapy, some prescription medications (especially anticoagulants), severe liver disease, and some other serious diseases can lead to Vitamin K deficiency.

Vitamin K is synthesized by the body in the small intestine; Vitamin K is also found in some foods, but the Vitamin K content of most common foods is not known exactly. Because newborns cannot yet synthesize Vitamin K, and because breast milk is low in Vitamin K, newborns are sometimes given Vitamin K to prevent bleeding problems. Vitamin K is available only by prescription.

RDAS FOR VITAMIN K
Vitamin K is measured in micrograms (mcg). People who eat a normal diet generally ingest between 300 and 500 mcg daily.

RDAS FOR VITAMIN K	
Age in years	*Daily mcg*
birth to 6 months	5
6 months to 1	10
1 to 3	15
4 to 6	20
7 to 10	30
11 to 14	45
15 to 18 females	55
15 to 18 males	65
19 to 24 females	60
19 to 24 males	70
25+ females	65
25+ males	80
pregnant	65
nursing	65

DIETARY SOURCES OF VITAMIN K
Vitamin K is found in green, leafy vegetables such as spinach, broccoli, cabbage, turnip greens, lettuce, and kale. Small amounts of Vitamin K are in cheese, eggs, and liver.

CAUTIONS FOR VITAMIN K
If your doctor has prescribed Vitamin K for you, discuss potential problems with him or her. Generally, large amounts of Vitamin K are not toxic.

MINERALS

CALCIUM

What Calcium Does for You
Calcium is a mineral needed by the body to form healthy bones and teeth and for the proper functioning of the heart, muscles, and nervous system. The average adult male body contains nearly 3 pounds of calcium. A serious deficiency of calcium leads to osteoporosis, or the loss of calcium from the bones. This makes the bones thin and easily broken. Osteoporosis is a particular problem for older women because their bodies absorb less calcium after menopause.

Supplemental calcium is sometimes recommended for pregnant and nursing women. Calcium in supplements is usually in the form of a calcium salt such as calcium carbonate or calcium lactate. The amount of usable calcium (also called elemental calcium) varies among the different salts. Calcium carbonate tablets generally have the most usable calcium.

RDAS FOR CALCIUM
Vitamin D is necessary for the proper absorption of calcium in the small intestine. A diet deficient in Vitamin D may also be deficient in calcium. The adult RDA for calcium is 800 milligrams (mg). Some researchers and doctors feel that a higher RDA for older women may help prevent osteoporosis. They suggest an RDA of 1,000 mg for premenopausal women and 1,500 mg for postmenopausal women. The National Research Council, however, has not changed its recommendations. Calcium in measured in milligrams (mg).

RDAS FOR CALCIUM	
Age in years	*Daily mg*
birth to 6 months	400
6 months to 1	600
1 to 10	800
11 to 24	1,200
25+	800
pregnant	1,200
nursing	1,200

DIETARY SOURCES OF CALCIUM
Calcium is found in dairy products such as low-fat milk, low-fat cheese, and low-fat yogurt. Butter, cream, and other fatty dairy products do not have much calcium. Dark green leafy vegetables such as kale, spinach, bok choy, and collard greens are high in calcium. Other good vegetable sources of calcium include broccoli, beans, dried apricots, and whole-grain products. Calcium is also found in shrimp, in canned fish that includes the bones (salmon, sardines, and the like), and in tofu and oranges.

CAUTIONS FOR CALCIUM
Very large doses of calcium (more than 3 grams daily) could interfere with the metabolization of other vitamins and minerals. If your doctor has prescribed calcium for you, discuss potential problems with him or her.

IODINE

What Iodine Does for You

Iodine is a mineral that is crucial for the formation of thyroid hormones, which help regulate the body's metabolism. The primary symptom of iodine deficiency is goiter, or enlargement of the thyroid gland in the neck. Goiter was once a widespread problem, but the introduction of iodized table salt in 1924 caused the incidence of goiter to drop sharply in the United States. Today, most cases of goiter are not related to a lack of iodine.

RDAS FOR IODINE

Iodine is essential for the body, but only very small amounts are needed. Excess iodine is excreted in the urine. Iodine is measured in micrograms (mcg).

RDAS FOR IODINE	
Age in years	*Daily mcg*
birth to 6 months	40
6 months to 1	50
1 to 3	70
4 to 6	90
7 to 10	120
11+	150
pregnant	175
nursing	200

DIETARY SOURCES OF IODINE

Iodine is found primarily in iodized salt, shellfish, and seafood. One teaspoon of iodized salt contain 420 mcg of iodine; thus most people will get more than enough iodine from a normal diet. Sea salt does not contain iodine. Some bakery breads also contain iodine because it is used as dough stabilizer.

CAUTIONS FOR IODINE

Iodine intake as large as 2 milligrams (mg) a day causes no toxicity in adults. Too much iodine is not the cause of hyperthyroidism.

IRON

What Iron Does for You

Iron is a mineral needed by the body to produce healthy red blood cells. Iron deficiency can lead to anemia. This form of anemia is not uncommon in the United States. Iron deficiency can also be caused by prolonged bleeding caused by an ulcer or other problem. Pregnant women may need iron supplements.

RDAS FOR IRON

Iron is measured in milligrams (mg).

RDAS FOR IRON	
Age in years	*Daily mg*
birth to 6 months	6
6 months to 1	10
1 to 10	10

11 to 18 male	12
19+ male	10
11 to 50 female	15
51+ female	10
pregnant	30
nursing	15

DIETARY SOURCES OF IRON

Iron is found in organ meats such as liver, red meat, fish, and poultry. Vegetable sources of iron include beans, peas, dried fruits, dark green leafy vegetables such as spinach, strawberries, blackberries, broccoli, wheat germ, whole grains, and nuts. Many grain, cereal, and bakery products are fortified with iron.

The human body does not absorb iron well. Meat contains heme iron, which absorbed more readily than the iron in plant foods. Eating foods rich in Vitamin C at the same time helps improve iron absorption.

CAUTIONS FOR IRON

Iron toxicity is very rare. If your doctor has prescribed iron for you, discuss the proper way to take the medicine and any potential problems with him or her.

MAGNESIUM

What Magnesium Does for You

Magnesium is a mineral needed for the proper functioning of many complex body processes, including many also regulated in part by calcium. Magnesium deficiency is sometimes found in people with diabetes, kidney disease, and serious illnesses, especially those affecting the digestive system. Severe magnesium deficiency is rarely seen.

RDAS FOR MAGNESIUM

Excess magnesium is excreted by the body in the urine. Magnesium is measured in milligrams (mg).

RDAS FOR MAGNESIUM	
Age in years	*Daily mg*
birth to 6 months	40
6 months to 1	60
1 to 3	80
4 to 6	120
7 to 10	170
11 to 14 female	280
11 to 14 male	270
15 to 18 female	300
15 to 18 male	400
19+ females	280
19+ males	350
pregnant	320
nursing	280

DIETARY SOURCES OF MAGNESIUM

Magnesium is found in many foods. Milk and seafood are good animal sources of magnesium. Good vegetable sources of magnesium include nuts, peanuts, beans, peas, whole grains, green leafy vegetables, bananas, and avocados.

CAUTIONS FOR MAGNESIUM

People with kidney problems or kidney failure may develop magnesium toxicity.

PHOSPHORUS

What Phosphorus Does for You

Phosphorus is a mineral needed build strong bones and teeth and help the body function normally in many other ways. Phosphorus is found in all plant and animal foods. Phosphorus deficiency is almost impossible, but some people who take large amounts of aluminum hydroxide antacids for a long time may develop phosphorus deficiency.

RDAS FOR PHOSPHORUS

Exactly how much phosphorus the human body needs is unknown. The National Research Council sets the RDA at the same levels as calcium. Phosphorus is measured in milligrams (mg).

RDAS FOR PHOSPHORUS	
Age in years	*Daily mg*
1 to 10	800
11 to 24	1,200
25+	800
pregnant	1,200
nursing	1,200

DIETARY SOURCES OF PHOSPHORUS

Phosphorus is found in virtually all plant and animal foods. Protein-rich foods such as milk, meat, poultry, and fish are good sources of phosphorus, as are beans, peas, lentils, nuts, and grains.

CAUTIONS FOR PHOSPHORUS

Very high doses of phosphorus may cause problems related to lowering the calcium level in the blood.

SELENIUM

What Selenium Does for You

Selenium is a mineral that is essential as an antioxidant. Free radicals (unattached oxygen molecules) in the body can oxidize, or damage, cells in the body. Selenium helps prevent this from happening. Selenium and Vitamin E work closely together; a deficiency of one often also means a deficiency of the other. The importance of selenium in the diet was not proven until 1979.

RDAS FOR SELENIUM

Only very small amounts of selenium are needed. Selenium is measured in micrograms (mcg).

RDAS FOR SELENIUM

Age in years	Daily mcg
birth to 6 months	10
6 months to 1	15
1 to 6	20
7 to 10	30
11 to 14 male	40
11 to 14 female	45
15 to 18	50
19+ male	70
19+ female	55
pregnant	65
nursing	75

DIETARY SOURCES OF SELENIUM

Selenium is found in animal foods such as organ meats, poultry, and seafood. Plant foods can vary widely in their selenium content depending on the amount of selenium in the soil the plants grew in. Generally, whole grains are good sources of selenium.

CAUTIONS FOR SELENIUM

Selenium can be highly toxic in large doses. Doses up to three times the RDA are probably harmless but avoid exceeding the RDA.

ZINC

What Zinc Does for You

Zinc is a mineral needed for the proper functioning of many complex body processes, including digesting protein, forming enzymes, and maintaining the immune system. Zinc deficiency can cause loss of appetite, skin changes, slow wound healing, and immune system abnormalities. Children who eat a diet low in zinc tend to grow more slowly.

RDAS FOR ZINC

The body stores some zinc in the muscles and bones, but most excess zinc is eliminated through the intestines. Zinc is found in supplements in one of two forms: zinc sulfate or zinc gluconate. Both forms are well absorbed by the body, but zinc sulfate is more acidic and may cause stomach irritation in some people. Zinc is measured in milligrams (mg).

RDAS FOR ZINC

Age in years	Daily mg
birth to 1	5
1 to 10	10
11+ females	12
11+ males	15
pregnant	15
nursing, 1st 6 months	19
nursing, 2nd 6 months	16

DIETARY SOURCES OF ZINC

Zinc is found in animal foods such as meat, liver, poultry, eggs, and seafood. Zinc is also found in plant foods such as whole grain products. The zinc in plant foods is less accessible to the body than the zinc found in animal foods.

CAUTIONS FOR ZINC

Only a small amount more than the RDA of zinc (25 mg or more a day) can interfere with the body's use of copper. Larger doses of zinc over a long period can cause serious problems, including nausea, vomiting, and impairment of the immune system. Avoid exceeding the RDA for zinc.

TRACE MINERALS

The human body needs very small amounts, or traces, of other minerals in order to function properly—although researchers are still not sure about how or why many trace minerals affect the body. Trace minerals needed include aluminum, arsenic, boron, cadmium, chromium, copper, fluoride, lead, manganese, mercury, molybdenum, nickel, potassium, silicon, sodium, sodium chloride, sulfur, tin, and vanadium. In general, the amounts needed are so small that they are easily obtained from the diet and there is no need for supplementation.

POISON CONTROL CENTERS

ALABAMA
Regional Poison Control Center
Children's Hospital of Alabama
1600 Seventh Avenue South
Birmingham, AL 35233-1711
Emergency numbers:
800 292 6678
205 939 9201
205 933 4050

ARIZONA
TUCSON
Arizona Poison and Drug
    Information Center
Arizona Health Sciences Center
1501 North Campbell Avenue
Tucson, AZ 85724
Emergency numbers:
800 362 0101 (AZ only)
602 626 6016
PHOENIX
Samaritan Regional Poison Center
Good Samaritan Medical Center
1130 East McDowell Road
Phoenix, AZ 85006
Emergency number:
602 253 3334

CALIFORNIA
FRESNO
Fresno Regional Poison Control Center
Fresno Community Hospital
    and Medical Center
2823 Fresno Street
Fresno, CA 93715
Emergency number:
800 346 5922 (CA only)
LOS ANGELES
Los Angeles County Medical Association
    Regional Poison Control Center
1925 Wilshire Boulevard
Los Angeles, CA 90057
Emergency number:
213 484 5151

SAN DIEGO
San Diego Regional Poison Center
UCSD Medical Center
225 Dickinson Street
San Diego, CA 92103
Emergency numbers:
800 876 4766 (619 area code only)
619 543 6000
SAN FRANCISCO
San Francisco Bat Area Regional
        Poison Control Center
San Francisco General Hospital
1001 Potrero Avenue
San Francisco, CA 94110
Emergency numbers:
800 523 2222 (415 and 707 area codes only)
415 476 6600
SAN JOSE
Santa Clara Valley Medical Center
        Regional Poison Center
751 South Bascom Avenue
San Jose, CA 95128
Emergency numbers:
800 662 9886
408 299 5112
SACRAMENTO
UCDMC Regional Poison Control Center
2315 Stockton Boulevard
Sacramento, CA 95817
Emergency numbers:
800 342 9293 (CA only)
916 734 3692
ORANGE
UC Irvine Regional Poison Center
UCU Medical Center
101 The City Drive
Orange, CA 92668-3298
Emergency numbers:
800 544 4404 (southern CA only)
714 634 5988

COLORADO
Rocky Mountain Poison and Drug Center
645 Bannock Street
Denver, CO 80204-4507
Emergency numbers:
800 332 3073 (CO only)
303 629 1123

DISTRICT OF COLUMBIA
National Capital Poison Center
Georgetown University Hospital
3800 Reservoir Road, NW
Washington, DC 20007
Emergency numbers:
202 625 3333
202 784 4660 (TTY)

FLORIDA
Florida Poison Information Center
Tampa General Hospital
Box 1289
Tampa, FL
Emergency numbers:
800 282 3171 (FL only)
813 253 4444

GEORGIA
Georgia Poison Center
Grady Memorial Hospital
80 Butler Street, SE
Atlanta, GA 30335-3801
Emergency numbers:
800 282 5846 (GA only)
404 589 4400
404 525 3323 (TTY)

INDIANA
Indiana Poison Center
Methodist Hospital of Indiana
1701 North Senate Boulevard
Indianapolis, IN 46206
Emergency numbers:
800 382 9097
317 929 2323

KENTUCKY
Kentucky Regional Poison Center
of Kosair Children's Hospital
Box 35070
Louisville, KY 40232-5070
Emergency numbers:
800 722 5725 (KY only)
502 629 7275

MARYLAND
Maryland Poison Center
20 North Pine Street
Baltimore, MD 21201
Emergency numbers:
800 492 2414 (MD only)
301 528 7701

MASSACHUSETTS
Massachusetts Poison Control System
300 Longwood Avenue
Boston, MA 02115
Emergency numbers:
800 682 9211 (MA only)
617 232 2120

MICHIGAN
DETROIT
Poison Control Center
Children's Hospital of Michigan
3901 Beaubien Boulevard
Detroit, MI 48201
Emergency number:
313 745 5711
GRAND RAPIDS
Blodgett Regional Poison Center
1840 Wealthy SE
Grand Rapids, MI 49506
Emergency numbers:
800 632 2727 (MI only)
800 356 3232 (TTY)

MINNESOTA
MINNEAPOLIS
Hennepin Regional Poison Center
Hennepin County Medical Center
701 Park Avenue
Minneapolis, MN 55415
Emergency numbers:
612 347 3141
612 337 7474 (TTY)
ST. PAUL
Minnesota Regional Poison Center
St. Paul-Ramsey Medical Center
640 Jackson Street
St. Paul, MN 55101
Emergency number:
612 221 2113

MISSOURI
Cardinal Glennon Children's Hospital
Regional Poison Center
1465 South Grand Boulevard
St. Louis, MO 63104
Emergency numbers:
800 366 8888
314 772 5200

MONTANA
Rocky Mountain Poison and Drug Center
645 Bannock Street
Denver, CO 80204-4507
Emergency number:
800 525 5042 (MT only)

NEBRASKA
The Poison Center
8301 Dodge Street
Omaha, NE 68114
Emergency numbers:
800 955 9119
402 390 5555

NEW JERSEY
New Jersey Poison Information
and Education System
201 Lyons Avenue
Newark, NJ 07112
Emergency number:
800 962 1253 (NJ only)

NEW MEXICO
New Mexico Poison and Drug
    Information Center
University of New Mexico
Albuquerque, NM 87131
Emergency numbers:
800 432 6866 (NM only)
505 843 2551

NEW YORK
LONG ISLAND
Long Island Regional Poison
    Control Center
Nassau County Medical Center
2201 Hempstead Turnpike
East Meadow, NY 11554
Emergency number:
516 542 2323

NEW YORK CITY
New York City Poison Control Center
455 First Avenue
New York, NY 10016
Emergency numbers:
212 POISONS
212 340 4494

OHIO
CINCINNATI
Regional Poison Control System
Cincinnati Drug and Poison
    Information Center
231 Bethesda Avenue
Cincinnati, OH 45267-0144
Emergency numbers:
800 872 5111
513 558 5111
COLUMBUS
Central Ohio Poison Center
Columbus Children's Hospital
700 Children's Drive
Columbus, OH 43205
Emergency numbers:
800 682 7625 (OH only)
614 228 1323
614 228 2272 (TTY)

OREGON
Oregon Poison Center
Oregon Health Sciences University
3181 SW Sam Jackson Park Road
Portland, OR 97201
Emergency numbers:
800 452 7165 (OR only)
503 494 8968

PENNSYLVANIA
PHILADELPHIA
The Poison Control Center
One Children's Center
34th and Civic Center Boulevard
Philadelphia, PA 19104
Emergency number:
215 386 2100
PITTSBURGH
Pittsburgh Poison Center
3705 Fifth Avenue
Pittsburgh, PA 15213
Emergency number:
412 681 6669

RHODE ISLAND
Rhode Island Poison Center
Rhode Island Hospital
593 Eddy Street
Providence, RI 02902
Emergency number:
401 277 5727

TEXAS
North Texas Poison Center
Box 35926
Dallas, TX 73235
Emergency numbers:
800 441 0040 (TX only)
214 590 5000

UTAH
Intermountain Regional Poison Control Center
50 North Medical Drive
Salt Lake City, UT 84132
Emergency numbers:
800 456 7707 (UT only)
801 581 2151

VIRGINIA
Blue Ridge Poison Center
UVA-Blue Ridge Hospital
Box 67
Charlottesville, VA 22901
Emergency numbers:
800 451 1428
804 925 5543

WEST VIRGINIA
West Virginia Poison Center
West Virginia University Health Sciences Center
3110 MacCorkle Avenue, SE
Charleston, WV 25304
Emergency numbers:
800 642 3625 (WV only)
304 348 4211

WYOMING
The Poison Center
8301 Dodge Street
Omaha, NE 68114
Emergency numbers:
800 955 9119
402 390 5555

INDEX